Loving Someone with Tourette Syndrome

A Partner's, Parent's, and Family Member's Guide to Tics, Premonitory Urges, Co-Occurring OCD/ADHD, and Building a Calm, Connected Home

Patrick Nathaniel Marsh

This book is intended for general informational and educational purposes only. It does not constitute medical, psychological, psychiatric, legal, or professional advice of any kind, and it is not a substitute for professional evaluation, diagnosis, or treatment. Readers who have concerns about their own health or the health of a family member should consult a qualified healthcare provider.

The information in this book reflects the author's research and interpretation of publicly available sources as of the time of writing. Clinical guidelines, research findings, and recommended treatments may change. The author and publisher make no representations or warranties, express or implied, about the completeness, accuracy, or suitability of the information contained herein. No guarantee of results is offered or implied.

All named characters, composite case examples, and illustrative scenarios in this book are fictional constructs used for educational purposes. Any resemblance to actual persons, living or dead, is entirely coincidental and unintentional. No individual, organisation, or clinical practice has been identified in ways intended to harm or misrepresent them. Readers are solely responsible for their own choices and actions in response to the material in this book.

First Edition:2026

ISBN: 978-1-7646815-0-6

Table of Contents

Preface

The clinical understanding of Tourette Syndrome has advanced considerably in the past two decades. The identification of the premonitory urge as a neurologically distinct feature of tic generation, the development and validation of Comprehensive Behavioral Intervention for Tics as a first-line treatment, and the growing body of research on what clinicians now call the TS-Plus profile have together produced a substantially more detailed picture of the condition than existed a generation ago. What has not kept pace with this clinical progress is the translation of that knowledge into resources for the people who live most closely with someone who has Tourette Syndrome.

Tourette Syndrome is a neurodevelopmental condition characterised by involuntary motor and vocal tics, onset in childhood, and a strong association with co-occurring conditions including attention-deficit/hyperactivity disorder, obsessive-compulsive disorder, and anxiety. The condition is not rare: current estimates place prevalence at roughly one in one hundred school-age children. What distinguishes Tourette Syndrome from the public understanding of it, shaped primarily by media portrayals fixated on its least common feature, is the degree to which the tics are only one part of a considerably larger clinical picture.

The gap this book fills is specific. Partners, parents, and siblings of people with Tourette Syndrome routinely navigate the condition without adequate information. They misread suppression rebound as intentional behaviour. They respond to premonitory urges with requests for voluntary control that are neurologically impossible to honour. They accommodate OCD in ways that maintain rather than reduce it. They approach school meetings without knowledge of the legal frameworks that govern accommodation. They enter treatment conversations without a working understanding of the evidence hierarchy that places CBIT above medication as a first-line recommendation. None of these errors are failures of care. They are failures of available information. This book addresses that failure directly.

The book applies a framework built around four functions: neurological understanding, which replaces blame and confusion with accurate knowledge; relational competence, which translates that knowledge into communication and household strategies; systems advocacy, which equips family members to secure appropriate support in educational and workplace settings; and caregiver sustainability, which addresses the family member's own experience as a variable with direct consequences for household function. Each chapter is structured around a clear principle, grounded in the current research literature, and closed with a specific action step.

This book is the eighth title in the publisher's "Loving Someone with..." series, which examines the family caregiver experience across a range of chronic and neurodevelopmental conditions. Where the series typically addresses either a clinical population or an emotional experience, this title is distinguished by its dual commitment to clinical accuracy and practical application within a single volume. It does not assume clinical training on the part of the reader, nor does it simplify the research to the point of inaccuracy.

The primary audience is partners, parents, and adult siblings of people with Tourette Syndrome or persistent tic disorders. Adults with TS who wish to share a structured, clinically grounded resource with family members will find the book equally useful. Healthcare providers seeking a lay-accessible companion to clinical treatment may also find it a practical referral resource.

This book does not offer a cure, a guaranteed improvement in tic severity, or a replacement for professional evaluation and treatment. It offers something more durable: the knowledge to stop making things inadvertently worse and the tools to start making them measurably better. That is what an informed family member can do, and it is more than most families have been given the means to attempt.

Introduction You Are Not Failing

There was a night when Margot sat in her car in the driveway for twenty-two minutes before going inside. She did not know how long she had been sitting there until she checked her phone. The street was quiet. The lights in her front window were warm and ordinary-looking, and she sat with both hands in her lap and told herself she just needed one more minute before she walked in.

She loved her son. She had loved him since before he was born and she had not stopped loving him once in the eleven years since. That was not the question. The question was whether she was going to say the wrong thing again at the dinner table, whether her face was going to do the thing it did when the sounds started, whether tonight she was going to handle it the way a good mother should handle it rather than the way she kept actually handling it. She sat in the car and breathed and then she went inside.

Margot is not unusual. In the communities built around Tourette Syndrome, on the forums and in the support groups and in the quiet conversations that happen between partners at the end of long days, the same exhaustion appears again and again. It wears different faces. It shows up as the parent who has read every website and still does not understand why pointing out the tics seems to make them worse. It shows up as the partner who wonders whether they are making things harder by trying so hard to make things easier. It shows up as the spouse who has learned to manage the visible symptoms reasonably well but is blindsided, repeatedly, by the rage or the OCD or the sleepless nights, none of which anyone mentioned when the diagnosis was handed over.

The exhaustion is real. The confusion is real. And neither one of them means you are failing.

What they mean, almost without exception, is that you did not have the right information. Not because you were careless or inattentive, but because the right information for family members of people with Tourette Syndrome has simply not been written down in one place before. There are books for the person with TS. There are clinical guides for the professionals who treat them. There are memoirs, and there are academic papers, and there are websites that answer one question at a time. But there has not been a book written for you.

This is that book.

What This Book Is For

This book was written for the partner who shares a bed with someone whose body will not be still. For the parent who sits across the dinner table and does not know where to look. For the sibling who has spent years simultaneously defending and feeling ashamed of the same person. For the adult child of someone with TS who is only now, years later, beginning to make sense of what growing up in that house was like.

The problem this book is designed to solve is not Tourette Syndrome itself. You cannot solve Tourette Syndrome, and this book will not pretend otherwise. The problem it is designed to solve is the gap between how much you love someone and how little you know about what they are actually experiencing. That gap is where most of the damage happens. That gap is where the dinner table arguments start, and where the resentment builds quietly over months, and where the person with TS gradually learns that home is not as safe as it should be. Closing that gap, even partially, changes everything.

What You Will Find Here

This book moves in a specific direction. It begins with neuroscience, not because you need to become a neurologist, but because understanding what a tic actually is, in the most straightforward terms possible, is the single most useful piece of information a family member can have. From there, it builds toward the full picture of what clinicians call TS-Plus, which is the reality that most people with Tourette Syndrome also live with ADHD, OCD, anxiety, and a handful of other conditions that nobody warned you about. Then it turns practical. Communication scripts. Treatment decisions. School accommodations. The caregiver's own experience, which matters too.

Each chapter ends with something you can do. Not something vague, not a general encouragement to reflect, but a specific action that can shift one small thing in the right direction. Small shifts, applied consistently, are how families like yours change.

A Note on How to Read This Book

Some readers will go straight through. Others will turn immediately to the chapter that matches the thing that happened last week. Both approaches work. If you are in the middle of a crisis, the chapter on communication scripts may be where you need to begin. If you are newly navigating a diagnosis, start at the beginning and let the understanding build.

If you are reading this alongside the person you love, some chapters will be easier to share than others. The chapter on what TS actually feels like from the inside may be a good one to read together. The chapter on the mistakes families make is probably better read alone first.

One last thing before you begin. The five mistakes described in Chapter 4 are not a list of accusations. They are the mistakes made by almost every family that enters this experience without a guide. If you recognize yourself in all five of them, that is not evidence that you are a bad partner or parent. It is evidence that you needed information and did not have it. You have it now.

Self-Assessment: Which Mistakes Do You Recognize?

Before reading further, read through the five patterns below and note which ones feel familiar. There is nothing to score and no wrong answer. This is a starting point, not a verdict.

First: drawing attention to tics when they happen, either by commenting on them, asking about them, or reacting visibly. Second: asking the person with TS to try to hold back or stop their tics, particularly in social situations. Third: rearranging significant parts of daily family life to prevent or avoid tic triggers, in ways that reduce rather than support the person with TS. Fourth: explaining the diagnosis to every teacher, relative, or stranger who might notice, without checking whether the person with TS wants that disclosure. Fifth: interpreting the behavioural effects of TS-related ADHD, OCD, or rage attacks as character flaws or deliberate choices.

Note which of these you recognise. You will find each of them examined, explained, and replaced with something more useful in the chapters ahead.

Chapter 1 Tics Are Never Chosen

The first year Eloise's daughter was in secondary school, the throat-clearing started. It was not dramatic, not at first. A small sound, slightly wet, repeated in loose clusters throughout the day. Eloise noticed it on a Thursday at dinner and by Friday she had found herself saying, gently, across the pasta, "Sweetheart, can you try not to do that?" Her daughter looked at her. The sound came again almost immediately, louder this time. Eloise said nothing and finished her meal and told herself she would handle it differently next time.

She did not handle it differently next time.

For three months, Eloise tracked the sound the way you track a dripping tap. She became exquisitely aware of its timing and frequency. She tried several strategies: the gentle reminder, the raised eyebrow, the firm request, the conversation about how other people might perceive it. Her daughter grew quieter at the table, then quieter in the car, then quieter in the house generally. The tic did not improve. The relationship did.

It was a school nurse, during a routine appointment, who first used the word Tourette. The nurse mentioned premonitory urge, which Eloise had never heard, and said something about how asking someone to stop a tic was a little like asking someone not to sneeze after they had already felt the tickle. Eloise drove home with her daughter and pulled over on a residential street three blocks from their house and sat for a moment. She had spent three months trying to extinguish a sneeze.

The chapter principle follows from this story because the principle follows from this reality. Understanding that tics are not choices is not a soft or sentimental point. It is a clinical fact that changes the way families behave, and the way families behave changes what home feels like for the person with TS. If you absorb only one thing from this entire book, let it be this: the tic is not a decision. It never was.

The Pressure That Must Release

A tic is a sudden, rapid, recurrent, non-rhythmic movement or sound. It can be a blink, a shoulder shrug, a head jerk, a throat clear, a sniff, a word, a phrase, or a combination of several of these in sequence. What distinguishes a tic from a habit or a mannerism is not how it looks from the outside but what is happening on the inside, and that inside experience is where most family members begin to go wrong.

Researchers who study TS have established that the majority of people with the condition, somewhere between 80 and 90 percent of adults and many children by middle childhood, experience what is called a premonitory urge before each tic (Leckman et al., 1993). The premonitory urge is a physical sensation, a building pressure or tension that gathers in the body, usually in the specific muscles or areas that are about to tic, and that demands release. People with TS describe it in various ways. An itch that has to be scratched. A pressure that builds until it must come out. A tight feeling that will not ease until the movement happens. A sensation like holding your eyes open when they want to close, but throughout the body.

The tic is the release of that pressure. When the tic happens, the urge resolves. When the tic is suppressed, the pressure does not resolve. It accumulates.

This matters for family members in a very specific way. When you ask someone with TS to stop ticking, you are not asking them to stop a behaviour. You are asking them to hold a sneeze that has already been triggered. They may be able to do it, briefly. But the sneeze is still there. And when it finally comes, it tends to come harder than it would have if it had been allowed to happen naturally.

Action challenge: For the next seven days, do not comment on, react to, or attempt to redirect any tic you observe. This is harder than it sounds, particularly if you have built habits around managing them. Keep a notebook nearby instead, and when you notice a tic, write down the time, what was happening in the environment, and whether the tics seemed to cluster or ease. You will learn more from this exercise than from any intervention.

The Hidden Cost of Holding Back

Elio was twenty-six when he started working in open-plan offices. Before that, he had studied from home through most of his undergraduate years, and before that, he had attended a school where his teachers had been briefed and where he had developed, over years of practice, a reasonable ability to suppress his most visible tics during lessons. He was good at it. He had no idea what it cost him.

The suppression cost in Tourette Syndrome is one of the most consistently reported features of the condition, and one of the most consistently misunderstood by the families of people who live with it. When someone with TS spends a day at school or at work suppressing their tics, they are expending significant mental and physical energy. The effort is not trivial. It is sustained, effortful, and tiring in ways that are difficult to explain to someone who has never felt a premonitory urge.

Research confirms that suppression is possible for many people with TS, but that it comes at a cost. Studies using laboratory conditions have shown that people who suppress tics in one period are significantly more likely to show increased tic activity in the period immediately following, a phenomenon called rebound (Himle et al., 2007)., this rebound typically happens at home, in the evening, after school or work. The person with TS walks through the door and the tics that were held back all day come out in a rush. They may tic more intensely at home than they do anywhere else.

Many parents and partners interpret this wrongly. They see the tic intensity at home and conclude that the TS is severe, or worsening, or that their home is somehow making things worse. In fact, the opposite may be true. The tic release at home often means the person with TS feels safe there. It means they trust the home environment enough to let the pressure out. The problem arises only when family members respond to this release with the same corrective strategies they have been applying all along, strategies which, as we have seen, do not work and tend to make things worse.

Elio did not understand why he fell apart every evening until a therapist explained suppression cost in a single conversation. He had attributed his evening tic surges to stress, to screens, to diet, to a dozen other things. What was actually happening was much simpler. He had been holding the sneeze all day, and when he got home, it came out.

Action challenge: Ask the person with TS in your life, in a low-stakes moment, what the end of a school or work day feels like. Do not offer interpretations. Ask only questions, and listen to the answers. You may find that what you have been interpreting as behaviour directed at you has nothing to do with you at all.

Why Stress Turns Up the Volume

Sebastian's tics had been manageable since he was fourteen. Mild. Mostly invisible to people who did not know what to look for. His partner of three years, Lucia, had almost forgotten they were there until the year Sebastian changed jobs, moved cities, and lost a parent within six months. That year, the tics came back in a way that felt, to Lucia, like a new condition entirely. She wondered whether he had developed something different. She wondered whether the move had somehow caused it. She wondered whether she was somehow contributing.

None of those things were true. What was true was that stress, anxiety, and fatigue are among the most reliably documented tic modulators in the research literature (Findley, 2001; Conelea & Woods, 2008). When the nervous system is under sustained load, tic frequency and intensity tend to increase. When the person with TS is anxious, the premonitory urges arise more often and more forcefully. When they are tired, the suppression effort that usually keeps tics contained becomes too costly to sustain.

The practical implication for families is important. When tics increase, the instinct is to look for what changed and try to fix it. This is a reasonable instinct, but it points in the wrong direction when it focuses on the tics themselves rather than the underlying nervous system load. A partner who reduces external pressure, creates predictable routines, and resists the urge to add their own anxious monitoring to an already overloaded system is doing something genuinely useful. A partner who responds to increased tics with increased observation and increased commentary is adding weight to an already strained structure.

This is not an argument for silence or for pretending nothing is happening. It is an argument for understanding what is happening before deciding how to respond. When tics increase, the most useful question is not "what is causing these tics" but "what is the overall load on this person's nervous system, and what can I do to reduce it."

Lucia took three months to reach this understanding, and she reached it only after a paediatrician said something in an appointment that she wrote down on the back of a receipt and kept in her wallet. The note said: calm the system, not the tic. She still has it.

The Iceberg Nobody Shows You

A neurologist named Oscar once used an analogy with the parents of a twelve-year-old that is worth passing on. He held up one finger and said: the tic is this much of what is happening. Then he spread both arms wide and said: the rest of it is this much of what is happening. The parents had come in focused entirely on the finger.

The iceberg metaphor for Tourette Syndrome refers to a simple clinical truth. The tics are visible. They are the part of TS that other people see and comment on and react to. But tics are, for most people with TS, not the most impairing part of the condition. What sits below the waterline, unseen, is often far larger: the premonitory urges, the suppression effort, the mental vigilance in social settings, the shame that accumulates over years of being stared at or corrected, the fatigue that comes from carrying all of this without being able to explain it.

Understanding the iceberg does not require a medical degree. It requires only a shift in where you look. When you see a tic, the tic is the surface event. Beneath it is a person managing an internal experience that they have likely been managing alone, mostly without language for it, since early childhood. The appropriate response to that is not correction. It is curiosity, and where possible, steadiness.

Families who shift from correcting the visible tip to attending to the full experience of the person with TS find that their relationships change considerably. Not because the tics change, but because the person with TS stops bracing for the correction that used to come with every cluster of movement.

Summary

A tic is the release of a premonitory urge, a physical pressure that builds before each tic and resolves when the tic occurs. Suppression is possible for many people with TS but comes at a real cost, including rebound at home and increased fatigue. Stress, anxiety, and exhaustion raise tic frequency and intensity consistently. Telling someone to stop ticking does not reduce tics; it redirects the pressure and increases the physical and emotional cost. The visible tic is a small fraction of the total experience. The family members who help most are the ones who understand the invisible remainder.

Chapter 2 More Than the Tics

Felix had been managing his Tourette Syndrome for most of his life. He had told his partner Valeria about it on their fourth date, the same way he told everyone, matter-of-factly, after a tic made it impossible to pretend otherwise. Valeria had taken it in stride. She had grown up with a cousin who had a movement disorder and she thought she understood what she was accepting. The blinking, the occasional shoulder roll, the sniff that came when he was anxious. She understood those things. She was prepared for those things.

She was not prepared for what happened on a Sunday afternoon eight months into living together, when Felix could not find his keys. He had left them somewhere in the apartment and he knew he had left them somewhere in the apartment and he had been over every surface twice and then three times and then four times before Valeria offered to help, and he said in a voice she had never heard before that he did not need help, he needed to find his keys in the specific way that he needed to find his keys, and could she please not touch anything. She stood very still. The apartment was small and suddenly felt smaller.

Valeria knew about the tics. She did not know about the OCD. She did not know, because nobody had told her, that the majority of people with Tourette Syndrome also live with at least one other condition, usually several, and that those conditions can be more disruptive to daily life than the tics themselves. She had been given one piece of the picture and assumed it was the whole thing.

This is one of the most common and most costly misunderstandings in TS families. The tics are visible and named and, after a period of adjustment, manageable as a concept. The rest of`the picture arrives without warning. Understanding it in advance, before the Sunday afternoon with the keys, is what this chapter is designed to provide.

The principle here is this: Tourette Syndrome is rarely a single-condition diagnosis. Most people with TS live with what clinicians now call TS-Plus, a constellation of co-occurring conditions that includes ADHD, OCD, anxiety, rage attacks, sleep disruption, and depression in various combinations and intensities. The tics are the part of TS that gets named. The rest is what the family lives with every day.

ADHD Is Not Bad Behavior

The most common co-occurring condition in Tourette Syndrome is attention-deficit/hyperactivity disorder. Research consistently finds ADHD present in between 60 and 80 percent of people with TS, making it not an exception but a statistical expectation (Tourette Syndrome Association International Consortium for Genetics, 2007). This means that the majority of families navigating TS are simultaneously navigating the executive function difficulties, impulsivity, distractibility, and emotional dysregulation that characterise ADHD.

For family members, ADHD in TS presents a specific interpretive challenge. When a child with TS forgets their homework four days running, or leaves every cabinet open after getting a glass of water, or speaks before thinking in a way that causes hurt feelings, or loses track of a conversation mid-sentence, the family member faces a choice about how to frame what they are seeing. The choice is usually made unconsciously and is usually wrong.

The wrong framing is that this is carelessness, or disrespect, or a lack of effort. The correct framing is that this is executive function impairment, which is neurological in origin and not responsive to the same corrections that change deliberate behaviour. The distinction matters enormously because the family member's emotional response to the behaviour changes depending on how it is understood. Frustration at perceived carelessness is a different feeling from compassion for a neurological difficulty, and the family member's response to the person with TS will be different depending on which feeling is driving it.

Hugo was twenty-eight when he was finally assessed for ADHD, three years after his TS diagnosis. His partner Noemi had been describing him to her sister for those three years as brilliant but impossible to live with. After the assessment, she sat with the clinical report for a long time. She thought about the times she had accused him of not listening. She thought about the times she had cleaned the kitchen in silence with a pointed quality to her silence. She thought about the conversations that had ended badly because Hugo had interrupted her before she finished the sentence. She did not think these things to generate guilt. She thought them because the report had given her a new lens and she was adjusting it.

OCD in TS Wears Different Clothes

Obsessive-compulsive disorder is present in somewhere between 11 and 80 percent of people with Tourette Syndrome, with the wide range reflecting differences in how OCD is defined and measured across studies (Khalifa & von Knorring, 2005). What is consistently found is that OCD in the context of TS tends to present differently from OCD in the general population, and these differences matter for families.

Classic OCD, the kind most people have heard of, tends to centre on contamination fears, checking rituals, and harm obsessions. OCD in TS more commonly involves symmetry, incompleteness, "not just right" experiences, and a need to repeat actions until they feel correct (Miguel et al., 2000). Felix and his keys were a clear example of this. He was not afraid something would happen if he found the keys the wrong way. It was that finding them through any process other than the specific one his mind required would leave something unresolved in a way that felt unbearable.

The practical implication for family members is one that requires careful handling. When someone with TS-related OCD asks you to confirm something, to reassure them that a door is locked or that nothing bad will happen or that they did not say something wrong, the natural impulse is to provide the reassurance. It feels kind. It ends the question. It does not help.

Reassurance in OCD functions like scratching a mosquito bite. It relieves the discomfort immediately and temporarily, and makes the underlying problem worse over time. The itch comes back stronger and needs scratching sooner. Families who learn to respond to OCD reassurance requests with warmth but without the reassurance, a skill that can be developed with support from a therapist trained in exposure and response prevention, do significantly better in the long run than families who resolve each episode with reassurance and face a bigger episode the next day.

Action challenge: Notice, over the next two weeks, whether you have developed any regular reassurance patterns with the person with TS in your life. These might look like answering the same question multiple times, checking things on someone else's behalf, or confirming that situations are safe or acceptable more than once per incident. Write down what you notice. You do not need to change anything yet. First, see it clearly.

The Rage That Comes From Nowhere

Of all the features of TS-Plus, rage attacks are the most frightening for families and the least discussed in general resources. Research estimates rage attacks in somewhere between 25 and 70 percent of people with TS, with most estimates clustering around 37 to 50 percent (Budman et al., 2000). Despite this, they are often not mentioned at the time of diagnosis, leaving families unprepared for an experience that can feel, when it happens, like something has gone catastrophically wrong with the person they love.

A TS-related rage attack is not a temper tantrum and it is not evidence of underlying violence. It is a neurologically-driven explosion of emotional and physical intensity that typically rises very fast, peaks, and then resolves, often leaving the person with TS exhausted and genuinely remorseful. The triggers tend to be small, disproportionate to the intensity of the response. A question asked at the wrong moment. An interruption. A minor frustration encountered at the end of a long day of suppression. The attack looks like rage. What is driving it is a nervous system that has been under sustained pressure and has exceeded its capacity for modulation.

Clara's son Martin was nine when the first rage attack happened. She had asked him to put on his shoes. He had been ticcing heavily all afternoon after a school day, and when she asked about the shoes, something in him simply went. He was not angry at her. He was not angry about the shoes. What happened in the next ninety seconds was loud and intense and over before she could process it, and afterwards he cried and said he was sorry and did not seem to understand what had happened either. Clara called the paediatrician the next morning and described what had happened. The paediatrician said: that is consistent with what we see in TS. Clara wrote that down and stared at it for a while.

Understanding rage attacks as neurological rather than behavioural does not make them easier to experience in the moment. It does make it easier to respond to them effectively rather than reactively, and it makes the repair conversation afterwards much more productive for everyone involved.

Sleep Anxiety and the Night Hours

Sleep difficulties in Tourette Syndrome are documented in between 12 and 62 percent of people with the condition, with the range reflecting different definitions of sleep problems across different studies (Ghosh et al., 2014). What families observe is often a combination of factors. Some people with TS continue to tic during lighter stages of sleep, which can disrupt their own rest and the rest of their sleeping partners. Many people with TS have co-occurring anxiety that makes it difficult to fall asleep in the first place. Those who also have ADHD may have delayed sleep phase issues, meaning their natural sleep timing is shifted later, which creates conflict with school and work schedules.

For family members, the practical effects of TS-related sleep disruption can extend far beyond bedtime. A person with TS who has not slept well will typically tic more, regulate their emotions less effectively, and have less executive function capacity the following day. The morning may therefore be a disproportionately difficult time for the whole household, not because of anything that happened in the morning, but because of what happened the night before.

Recognising this connection, between the quality of the previous night and the quality of the next day, gives families something genuinely useful to work with. Predictable sleep routines, reduced screen exposure in the hours before bed, and sleep environments that are as comfortable and low-stimulus as possible are all supported by the research on TS-related sleep (Ghosh et al., 2014). These are not dramatic interventions. They are the small adjustments that reduce overall system load in ways that accumulate over time.

Seeing the Whole Picture

The TS-Plus checklist at the end of this chapter is not a diagnostic tool. It is a starting point. Its purpose is to help family members look at the full picture of what the person with TS in their life is experiencing, rather than the single piece that was named at diagnosis.

If you read through the descriptions of ADHD, OCD, rage attacks, sleep disruption, anxiety, and depression in this chapter and recognised your family member in more than two or three of them, that recognition is valuable. Take it to your next medical appointment. Name what you have observed. Ask whether the full TS-Plus profile has been assessed. Many families spend years addressing one piece of a much larger picture because no one took the time to map the whole thing.

Valeria, eventually, asked Felix if he would be willing to see a specialist who could assess the complete picture. He went. The assessment found TS, ADHD, and OCD, all moderately impairing, none of which had been formally identified beyond the TS diagnosis he had carried since he was twelve. He was, on the day of the assessment, thirty-one years old. He had been managing all three conditions with tools designed for one of them for nearly two decades.

Action challenge: Write down the five most challenging daily behaviours or patterns you observe in the person with TS in your life. Next to each one, note whether you have attributed it to the TS itself, to personality, or to something else. Then read the list again with the TS-Plus framework in mind. More than one of those behaviours may have a neurological explanation you have not yet been offered.

Summary

Most people with Tourette Syndrome also live with at least one significant co-occurring condition. ADHD is present in 60 to 80 percent of cases, bringing impulsivity, distractibility, and emotional dysregulation that can be mistaken for carelessness or bad attitude. OCD in TS often looks different from classic OCD, centering on symmetry and incompleteness rather than contamination fears. Rage attacks are common, neurologically driven, and not evidence of an underlying character problem. Sleep disruption is a consistent feature that shapes the entire following day. Seeing the full TS-Plus picture is not pessimistic; it is the beginning of accurate understanding.

Chapter 3 Life Inside the Tics

Hugo gave a talk at a small conference three years after his combined TS and ADHD diagnosis. He had agreed to speak on a panel about living with neurodevelopmental conditions in professional environments, and he had prepared what he thought was a solid fifteen-minute account of managing tics in the workplace. He had the statistics ready. He had the strategies. He had a clean narrative arc.

What he actually said, when he got to the microphone, was something he had not prepared. He said that the thing no one told him, the thing he had figured out only recently and only with help, was that he had been performing normality for so long that he had genuinely lost track of what it cost. He said that he arrived home every evening and he ticced more intensely than he did anywhere else and he had spent years interpreting this as a problem with his home life, as stress related to his relationship, as evidence that something was wrong with him at a level beneath the diagnosis. He said it had taken a very good therapist asking him a very simple question to understand that he was not falling apart at home. He was exhaling.

The audience was mostly clinicians and researchers. A woman in the third row, who turned out to be a parent, started crying before he had finished the sentence.

That moment is what this chapter is about. Not the clinical framework, though there is one. Not the research evidence, though there is that too. This chapter is about what it is actually like to be inside the experience that your family member is having, and why closing the gap between your understanding of that experience and their daily reality is the most important single shift available to you.

The principle is this: before any communication technique, any treatment decision, or any accommodation strategy can work, you need to understand what you are actually working with. The inner experience of Tourette Syndrome is not visible from the outside. The part that is visible, the tics, is often the least significant part of what the person with TS is managing. Understanding the hidden remainder does not mean you can fix it. It means you can stop accidentally making it worse.

The Never-Off Awareness

Consider what it would mean to spend every day in a state of constant, low-level physical vigilance. Not fear, not quite, but awareness. The awareness that your body may do something at any moment that will make other people notice you. The awareness that you are always being watched, or might be, and that the watching is always a little bit uncertain, sometimes curious, sometimes hostile, occasionally kind, but always uncertain and therefore always requiring monitoring.

This is the social vigilance that most people with TS develop during childhood and carry into adulthood as a fully formed and largely automatic system. It runs in the background of every interaction. Every meeting. Every meal out. Every classroom, every office, every waiting room. It is the continuous calculation of which environment is safe enough for which level of tic expression, which people in this room understand and which do not, how much suppression is required here, what the exit options are if suppression fails.

Research examining the quality of life of people with TS has consistently found that social functioning and self-esteem are more significantly affected than the tics themselves would predict (Eddy et al., 2011). In other words, the psychological load of managing social perception exceeds the physical load of the tics for many people. They are managing their bodies and they are managing other people's responses to their bodies and they are managing their own responses to other people's responses, all at the same time, every day.

For family members, the practical implication of understanding this is specific. When the person with TS arrives home and seems withdrawn, or irritable, or difficult to reach, the question worth asking is not "what did I do" or "what is wrong with them tonight." The question worth asking is: what were they managing today, and how much of it is still being carried?

Home as the Release Valve

One of the most reliably reported phenomena in qualitative research on TS is the difference in tic expression between home and public environments. People with TS tic more at home. They tic more in environments where they feel safe. They tic more with people they trust. This is not a malfunction. It is, on balance, a sign that the relationship and the environment are working correctly.

Coralie spent two years believing that something in her home environment was making her partner's TS worse. She had noticed, clearly and accurately, that her partner ticced more intensely in the evenings than during the day, more at weekends than during the week, more in the presence of close friends than in the presence of acquaintances. She had looked for triggers. She had considered whether her own anxiety was contagious. She had wondered whether she was doing something wrong.

She was not doing anything wrong. She was living with someone who had built, slowly and unconsciously, a graduated hierarchy of environments based on felt safety, and who placed their home at the top of that hierarchy. The tics at home were the tics that had been held back all day in environments further down the scale. They were not evidence of a problem at home. They were the evidence that home was where the holding stopped being necessary.

This reframe is not a small one. Once a family member understands that higher tic expression in their presence can indicate trust rather than trouble, the entire emotional weight of the home environment shifts. The tics stop being something that is happening to the family member and start being something that is happening in a relationship where enough safety has been built for that release to be possible.

The appropriate response to someone exhaling is not to tell them to hold their breath again.

Action challenge: Have one conversation this week with the person with TS in your life where the topic is what they need during the first hour after getting home. Not what would be polite or what you can offer, but what they actually need. Some people need quiet. Some need to be greeted normally and then left alone briefly. Some need physical contact and some need the opposite. You do not need to guess. You can ask.

The Shame That Grows in Silence

Oscar was seven when a teacher first told him to stop making noises in class. He did not know, at seven, that he could not stop. He knew only that the teacher had told him to stop and that he could not and that the other children had heard and that his face was hot. He had no language for what was happening. He had only the instruction to stop and the fact of his failure to stop and the eyes of the other children.

He is thirty-four now. He has a diagnosis, a therapist, a partner, and a job he likes. He still, when he catches someone looking at him during a tic, feels something close to what he felt at seven. He has described this to his partner in a single sentence that she has not forgotten: it is embarrassment that has been practised so many times it has become automatic.

Qualitative research examining the experience of people with TS across the lifespan has identified shame as a central and underaddressed feature (Conelea et al., 2013). This shame is not irrational. It is a response to years of living in a world that responds to the symptoms of Tourette Syndrome with staring, correction, laughter, imitation, and the countless smaller signals that communicate, reliably and repeatedly, that what is happening in your body is not acceptable.

For family members, understanding the cumulative weight of this shame changes the nature of certain conversations. When the person with TS in your life does not want to go to a particular event, or avoids a particular setting, or reacts disproportionately to what seems like a minor social misstep, the explanation may not be in the present moment. It may be in a pattern that started decades before they met you, a pattern of bracing for the response that always comes eventually.

You cannot undo that history. But you can decide what the response in your home looks and sounds like. And that is not a small thing.

What They Cannot Always Tell You

The language for living with TS from the inside is not widely available, and many people with TS, particularly those diagnosed in childhood before they had the conceptual tools to understand their own experience, have never developed it. They know what their body does. They know that it exhausts them. They know that certain environments are harder than others and that certain people make them feel safer and that some days are simply longer than others and they are not always sure why.

What they may not be able to tell you is the specific sequence: the urge, the decision to suppress, the accumulation of that effort over a day, the rebound that happens in the car on the way home. They may not have language for the fact that your reaction to their tics, even a reaction that consists only of a slight change in expression, registers. They may not be able to explain why the question "are you okay" asked in a certain tone during a tic cluster feels like something other than concern.

This is not a failure of the relationship. It is a feature of a condition that most people navigate largely alone, from childhood, without a guide. Part of what you can offer as a family member is the patience to ask questions over time and to build a shared vocabulary for the experience slowly, without requiring the full account to appear immediately.

Paloma's daughter was fourteen before she was able to explain to her mother that the tics at the dinner table were worse on the nights when the family talked about school. Not because school was a forbidden topic, but because the anticipation of being asked about homework triggered the anxiety that turned up the tic frequency, which triggered the self-consciousness, which triggered more anxiety, which triggered more tics. The chain was clear once she had the language for it. She had not had the language at seven, or ten, or twelve. At fourteen, with a therapist who had helped her map the sequence, she could finally say it.

Paloma sat with that conversation for a long time. She thought about all the school discussions at dinner over all those years and what they had actually been doing. Then she changed what the family talked about at dinner, and the difference was visible within a week.

Action challenge: Take fifteen minutes and write down, without judging it, every assumption you currently hold about why the person with TS in your life behaves the way they do in the moments that are hardest for you. Then, next to each assumption, write a question, not a rhetorical one, a real question you could ask them that might give you better information than the assumption. Keep the list. Use the questions when the time is right.

Summary

The inner experience of Tourette Syndrome includes constant social vigilance, the sustained effort of managing other people's responses to an involuntary body. Home is often the environment where tic expression is highest, because home is where suppression is no longer required, and higher tic expression at home is often a sign of safety rather than a sign of a problem. Shame accumulated over years of public exposure shapes how people with TS respond to social situations, including situations within their own families. The language for this inner experience develops slowly and often incompletely; the family member's patience in building shared understanding over time is one of the most genuinely useful things they can offer.

Chapter 4 Stop Making It Worse

The dinner table at the Delacroix household had a script that ran for two years without anyone naming it as a script. Zoe, the mother, would set the plates. Gabriel, her son, would sit down. A tic would happen, usually a head jerk or a sharp sniff, and Zoe would look up without meaning to. Then she would look down again, quickly, hoping he had not seen. He had always seen. Then one of two things would happen: she would say nothing and the silence would carry its own freight, or she would say something gentle and careful, something like "you okay, bud?", and he would say he was fine and mean, with the full force of a fourteen-year-old, that he was not fine and did not want to talk about it.

Zoe was not a careless parent. She read everything she could find. She attended a support group twice before deciding it was not the right fit. She kept her voice steady and her face as neutral as she could manage. She was trying, in the most earnest way possible, and the script kept running because she did not know it was a script. She did not know that looking up was a problem. She did not know that the gentle question was a version of the same problem. She had not been told.

She found out when a CBIT therapist, eight months into Gabriel's treatment, asked to spend forty minutes speaking with her alone. The therapist asked her what she typically did when Gabriel ticced at the dinner table. Zoe described the look and the question. The therapist said, gently, that both of those things were signalling to Gabriel's nervous system that the tic was an event worth responding to, which made the premonitory urge more likely to generate another tic, which made the sequence more likely to repeat. She said this was not Zoe's fault. She said it was, however, something Zoe could change.

The principle of this chapter is that love is not enough on its own, and that most families, without specific guidance, develop patterns of response to Tourette Syndrome that are well-intentioned and counterproductive. These patterns are not character flaws. They are natural responses to an unfamiliar situation that no one prepared you for. Naming them clearly, which is what this chapter does, is the beginning of changing them.

Drawing Attention Always Backfires

Attention is a tic amplifier. This is established in the research literature and has practical applications so direct that they can be stated as a rule: reduce attention directed at tics, including sympathetic attention, and you reduce the overall tic burden in the home environment (Conelea & Woods, 2008).

The forms of attention that amplify tics are broader than most family members expect. The obvious ones are direct: pointing out the tic verbally, asking whether the person with TS is aware of the tic, commenting on frequency or intensity. These are clearly attention-drawing and most family members learn to stop them relatively quickly.

The less obvious forms are where the persistent problem lives. An expression of visible concern during a tic cluster. A pause in conversation that tracks a tic. A facial adjustment, however controlled and however brief. Moving slightly away in a social setting when a tic occurs. Checking whether anyone else in the room noticed. All of these are read by the person with TS, who is almost certainly more attuned to the responses of those around them than you realise, and all of them signal that the tic is an event.

The corrective is not the elimination of all response. It is the development of what clinicians sometimes call neutral responding: maintaining the ordinary texture of interaction during tic clusters, continuing conversation, maintaining eye contact, and treating the tic as the background event it is rather than the foreground event it becomes when it receives attention.

This takes practice. Zoe found it took three weeks of consistent, deliberate effort before it began to feel natural. Gabriel noticed the change before she felt she had made one. He told her, on a Sunday, that dinner had been different lately, and she said she had been working on something, and he said, good.

The Suppression Request Is a Trap

The request for suppression, however gently framed, is among the most reliably documented exacerbators of tic activity in home environments. Research has shown consistently that voluntary suppression of tics is possible for many people with TS but results in a rebound period during which tic frequency and intensity increase beyond baseline levels (Himle et al., 2007). request suppression, particularly in high-stress social situations, they are repeatedly triggering the rebound cycle and increasing the total daily tic burden.

Beyond the physiological cost, the suppression request carries a relational cost that operates at a different level. Each request communicates, regardless of the words used, that the tic is a problem that the person with TS should manage better. Over years, these communications accumulate into a belief that is particularly damaging in adolescence and early adulthood, the period during which most people with TS are already doing the hardest work of making sense of their own neurology. The belief is: my body, as it naturally is, is not acceptable in the company of the people who love me most.

This is a belief worth going to some effort to prevent.

The alternative is not silence on the subject of tics. It is the development of a different conversation: one in which the family member's understanding of the premonitory urge and suppression cost is made explicit to the person with TS, in which the family member's behaviour changes to reflect that understanding, and in which the person with TS gradually learns, from experience rather than from words, that the tics are not a problem that must be managed for the family's comfort.

Action challenge: Consider the last time you asked the person with TS in your life to suppress, hold back, or try harder. Write down the situation. Write down what you were hoping to prevent. Then write down what you know now about the suppression cost and what that request actually did. This is not an exercise in self-criticism. It is an exercise in building new information into old situations so that the next situation can go differently.

When Help Becomes a Cage

Julian had been managing the grocery shopping alone for two years before he understood that this had started as an accommodation and had become a constraint. His partner Mateo had Tourette Syndrome and social anxiety, and the supermarket, with its fluorescent lighting and unpredictable encounters, had always been difficult. Julian had taken over the grocery shopping early in their relationship and it had felt like the right and kind thing to do.

What he had not accounted for was the slow contraction that happens when the world of a person with TS is gradually shaped by the avoidances of the people who love them. Mateo no longer went to the supermarket. He also no longer went to the cinema, which Julian had stopped suggesting because of the noise concern. He attended fewer family events, because Julian had quietly begun declining on his behalf when they seemed too complex. He had become, over two years of Julian's well-intended management, someone who did significantly less than he had done before, and neither of them had noticed when the line between support and restriction had been crossed.

There is a distinction in clinical work with TS families between accommodation and avoidance. Accommodation adjusts the environment or the process in ways that make participation possible. Avoidance eliminates the participation entirely. Both can look like support from the outside. Only one of them is.

Families who slip from accommodation into avoidance typically do so without any intention to restrict. They do it because restriction is easier in the moment than the alternative, which is tolerating the discomfort of watching someone they love navigate a difficult situation without rescuing them from it. The avoidance reduces discomfort now and reduces capability over time.

Julian and Mateo had a long conversation, eventually, in which Julian asked Mateo directly whether there were things he had stopped doing that he would like to start again. The list was longer than Julian had expected. Working through it took most of a year, one small re-entry at a time. Mateo now does the grocery shopping on Tuesday mornings, when the supermarket is quiet. It took four attempts before it stopped being difficult. Julian stayed home for all four and texted to check in without calling. The difference between those two choices, texting rather than calling, was one that Mateo had asked for specifically, and Julian had listened.

Telling Too Much Too Soon

Disclosure of a TS diagnosis is a clinical and personal decision that belongs to the person with TS, not to their family members. This sounds straightforward and is, in practice, one of the more complicated aspects of family life with TS.

Felix's mother had told his teachers, his coaches, his friends' parents, his extended family, and eventually, inadvertently, a stranger in a park that her son had Tourette Syndrome. She had done all of this with the intention of protecting him, of getting ahead of the tic before it confused or alarmed someone, of building him a network of informed and tolerant adults. What she had not understood was that each disclosure she made without his knowledge was a small removal of agency from a child who was already managing a significant loss of bodily agency. She was deciding, on his behalf, who got to know the most personal fact of his life and in what order and with what framing.

Felix did not understand, as a child, why he felt so uncomfortable at his coach's particular brand of hearty reassurance, or why the teachers' knowing looks made him feel conspicuous rather than supported. He understood, as an adult, that he had been managed by people who loved him in ways that had removed his ability to manage himself.

The rule of thumb that most TS clinicians offer to families is this: let the person with TS lead disclosure. Discuss together whether to tell a particular teacher, employer, or family member. Have the conversation about how much information to share and what language to use. Let the person with TS decide whether to be present for the disclosure conversation or to have it happen without them. The family member's role is to support this process, not to drive it.

There are exceptions, particularly with young children who do not yet have the understanding or the language to participate in disclosure decisions. In those cases, limited, purposeful disclosure to specific people with a direct need to know, such as a classroom teacher or a school nurse, is reasonable. The general announcement to everyone who might possibly notice is a different thing and serves the family member's anxiety more than the child's interest.

Behavior Is Not Character

The final and perhaps most persistent mistake made by families navigating TS-Plus is the attribution of the behavioural effects of ADHD, OCD, and rage attacks to character rather than neurology. This attribution is so common and so automatic that many family members make it hundreds of times before ever recognising it as a pattern.

When Martin left the cap off the toothpaste for the forty-third time, his mother Clara did not think: this is an executive function difficulty related to his ADHD. She thought: he is not paying attention. When he interrupted her mid-sentence, she did not think: the impulsivity in ADHD reduces the inhibitory control that allows most people to wait for the end of a sentence. She thought: he does not care what I am saying. When the keys situation happened with Felix, Valeria did not think: this is OCD presenting as a "not just right" experience requiring a specific sequence. She thought, for one terrible moment: who is this person.

All of these attributions are understandable. They are the attributions a person makes when they have one piece of the picture and are trying to interpret behaviour that does not fit the piece they have. The problem is not that the attributions are made in the moment. The problem is that they accumulate, quietly, into a persistent story about who the person with TS is, a story in which the neurological realities of their condition are read as evidence of how much they care or do not care, who they are trying to be, what they think of the people around them.

That story is wrong. The executive function impairment in ADHD is not a reflection of priorities. The compulsive behaviour in OCD is not a choice to impose on the household. The rage attack is not a decision to be frightening. Once these attributions are recognised and corrected, the relational dynamic shifts in ways that family members consistently describe as significant, even when the behaviour itself changes very little.

Action challenge: Over the next week, each time you find yourself interpreting a behaviour by the person with TS as evidence of what they think of you or how much they care about you, pause and ask one question: is there a TS-Plus explanation for this that I am not seeing? Write the behaviours and the alternative explanations down. You will begin to develop a new default lens, one that serves the relationship considerably better than the one you are currently using.

Summary

Five specific family behaviours consistently worsen tic severity or damage the relational fabric between family members and the person with TS. Drawing attention to tics, even sympathetic attention, amplifies tic frequency through the signal value that attention creates. Requesting suppression triggers the rebound cycle and communicates that the body as it naturally is must be managed for others' comfort. Replacing participation with avoidance appears supportive and gradually shrinks the world of the person with TS. Disclosing the diagnosis without the person with TS's involvement removes agency from someone who has already lost a significant amount of physical agency. Attributing neurological behaviour to character builds a false story that shapes the relationship for years. Each of these mistakes is reversible. Knowing they are mistakes is where the reversal begins.

Chapter 5 Say the Right Thing

Ines had memorised three sentences. She had written them on a notecard, kept the card in her wallet for two weeks, read it every morning before work, and rehearsed them in the shower until they stopped feeling strange in her mouth. The sentences were: "I see you. Take what space you need. I am right here." She had practised saying them in a calm, flat voice, without her hands moving, without the particular worried expression her face made when she was trying not to look worried.

She had been practising because the year before, when her husband Marcel had a tic attack in the car on the way to her sister's birthday dinner, she had done all the wrong things. She had pulled over. She had asked him what was wrong. She had reached across and touched his arm, which made it worse. She had said, in a voice she intended to be soothing, "It's okay, it's okay, it's okay," which is a thing people say when something is not okay and everyone in the car knows it. Marcel had ticced for eleven more minutes. They had missed the dinner. They had driven home in silence, and the silence had lasted three days.

The notecard was her attempt to not repeat that night.

The first time she used the three sentences was six weeks later, also in the car, also heading somewhere she cared about going. Marcel's neck began jerking, a cluster she recognised as the beginning of a significant episode. She said the three sentences. She did not pull over. She did not touch him. She kept her hands on the wheel and her eyes on the road and let the car stay moving and let him take the space the sentences had offered. The tic cluster lasted four minutes and then subsided. They made the event. They stayed for two hours. Driving home, Marcel said: "That was different. What you did. Thank you."

Ines said: "I practised."

What she had understood, in the two weeks of shower rehearsals and notecard mornings, was something that changes everything once it becomes clear: the right words, said badly, are still the wrong words. And the wrong words, said confidently and calmly, can do more damage than silence. Most family members in TS households have never been given a script. They have been left to improvise in the highest-pressure moments of daily life, with no preparation and no practice, and then wondered why the improvisation so often goes wrong.

Communication in TS families does not have to be improvised. The most useful responses can be learned, practised, and made automatic before they are needed. This chapter provides the material. The practice is yours to do.

The principle is this: in TS families, communication breaks down most reliably not from lack of love but from lack of prepared language. The right script, rehearsed in advance, is more useful than the most heartfelt improvisation in the moment.

Silence Is Sometimes the Script

The most counterintuitive communication lesson in TS families is that the most useful response during an acute tic episode is usually not words. It is steady presence without comment.

Research on the attention-tic relationship, which was introduced in Chapter 4, has direct applications for communication. Because attention amplifies tic severity, verbal responses during tic clusters, even well-intentioned ones, can extend the duration and intensity of the episode (Conelea & Woods, 2008). The "it's okay" offered by a worried family member carries a signal the person with TS reads immediately: this is being treated as an event. That reading alone is enough to increase premonitory urge intensity.

The alternative is not coldness. It is what Ines learned with her three sentences: brief, warm acknowledgement followed by a return to ordinary behaviour. The acknowledgement says: I see you, I am not alarmed, I am not going anywhere. The return to ordinary behaviour says: this is not a crisis, the conversation can continue, nothing has changed.

Ines's three sentences work because they do exactly this. They are not effusive. They do not ask questions. They do not offer reassurance in a way that signals distress. They state presence and then get out of the way.

For family members whose instinct is to manage acute moments verbally, learning to reduce words is harder than it sounds. The instinct to speak is the instinct to help, and it takes deliberate practice before silence and brief acknowledgement begin to feel like helping rather than abandoning. But the families who make this shift report consistent improvement in the duration and aftermath of tic episodes.

Action challenge: Write your own three-sentence script for the next time tics escalate in your presence. The sentences should acknowledge, not manage. They should be calm, short, and free of questions. Write them down. Read them aloud three times today, in a normal voice, as if you are actually saying them. Then put them somewhere you will see them tomorrow.

After the Storm Passes

The conversation that happens in the hours following a significant tic episode, a rage attack, or a public incident is one of the most important and most neglected communication moments in TS family life. It is the conversation that either builds something or quietly damages something, and most families have it badly.

The most common version goes like this. The episode ends. Everyone is tired. The family member who was affected by it most visibly wants to talk about what happened, and the person with TS wants the episode to stop being the subject. The family member interprets this as avoidance. The person with TS interprets the persistence as evidence that the family member cannot let things go. The conversation ends without resolution and starts again, in a slightly different form, three days later.

Marcel's experience of the post-episode conversation, before Ines developed her script, was that it always felt like a debrief he had not agreed to attend. Ines wanted to understand what had happened. Marcel understood what had happened. He had been there. He did not need to reconstruct it and he particularly did not need to do it while still fatigued from the episode.

What worked, once they found it, was the timed-delay conversation: a brief acknowledgement immediately after the episode, followed by a genuine choice about when to talk. "That looked hard. I am here whenever you want to talk about it. No rush." And then, genuinely, no rush. Not the studied patience that is actually impatience. Actual willingness to wait until the person with TS initiated.

This approach requires the family member to tolerate some uncertainty for longer than feels comfortable. It also tends to produce better conversations, because the person with TS enters them voluntarily rather than under pressure. Conversations chosen are more productive than conversations compelled.

Action challenge: Think of a recent episode that you attempted to process with the person with TS before they were ready. Write down what you said and what the response was. Then write an alternative opening that offers presence and choice rather than immediate processing. Practise that alternative until it comes naturally.

Talking About Treatment

The treatment conversation is the one most TS family members dread, and for understandable reasons. It carries the weight of everything that has been hard, all the appointments and disappointments and medication trials and behavioural setbacks, and it happens in the middle of an ongoing relationship where both people are tired and neither is entirely sure what the right answer is.

Noemi had been trying to raise the subject of CBIT with her partner Hugo for six months before she finally understood why the conversation kept failing. She was framing it as advocacy. He was hearing it as criticism. Every time she said something in the form of "I think we should try," he heard something in the form of "what you are doing is not enough." The conversation that would have helped them had been derailed, every time, by a framing problem.

The shift that helped was changing the subject of the sentence. Instead of "I think we should try a CBIT therapist," Noemi said: "I have been reading about CBIT. I want to understand it better. Would you be willing to read about it with me?" This is a different conversation. The subject is information rather than action. The invitation is to think together rather than to comply. And it does not carry the implicit criticism that the previous version always did.

Treatment conversations in TS families work better when they are framed as shared questions rather than proposals. "I am wondering about..." is a different entry point from "I think you should...". "What do you think about..." carries less pressure than "we need to talk about...". These are not merely diplomatic niceties. They change the actual structure of the conversation and the likelihood that the person with TS will engage rather than defend.

The research on CBIT family involvement suggests that family members who support treatment without directing it produce better outcomes than family members who drive the treatment process (Piacentini et al., 2010). This applies to treatment conversations as much as it applies to treatment itself.

Responding to OCD Without Feeding It

The OCD reassurance trap, introduced in Chapter 2, has a specific communication dimension that is worth addressing directly. The trap is that the natural language of reassurance, which sounds kind and produces short-term relief, is precisely the language that maintains and strengthens OCD over time.

Elio's partner Lucia had developed, over four years of living with his TS-related OCD, a fluent vocabulary of reassurance. She was good at it. She could answer the same question in twelve different ways, match her tone to the moment, and deliver the answer before he had finished asking. She did not know that every answer was making the next question more likely.

The alternative is not a refusal to engage. It is a different kind of engagement, one that acknowledges the distress without confirming the feared content. The structure looks like this: acknowledge the discomfort, name the OCD pattern, and redirect to the person's own capacity rather than external confirmation.

A practical script: "I can hear this feels hard right now. That sounds like OCD looking for certainty it will not get from me. You have handled this before." This is three things at once. It is warm, naming the feeling rather than dismissing it. It is accurate, naming the OCD dynamic without diagnosing in a way that sounds clinical or cold. And it is encouraging, pointing to past capacity without making false promises about the present moment.

This kind of response requires practice and will not feel natural at first. It is useful to develop it with a therapist trained in exposure and response prevention, so that the family member has support for what can be a difficult shift.

Scripts for the Extended Family

The conversation with grandparents, siblings, aunts, uncles, and family friends who do not understand TS is one of the most consistently reported stressors in TS family life. The people who love the family and who want to help, but who have been formed by the coprolalia stereotype, or who attribute tics to anxiety that could be resolved if the parents were firmer, or who offer well-intentioned advice that makes the person with TS feel like a problem to be solved.

Paloma had a mother-in-law named Margot who believed, with genuine and sincere conviction, that the tics would improve significantly if Paloma's son was given less screen time, more outdoor activity, and a stricter bedtime. Margot was not cruel. She was a product of a generation that had not encountered Tourette Syndrome as a neurological condition and a family that did not discuss medical matters in plain terms. She was also impossible to educate through argument, because argument was a form of disrespect to her and disrespect caused her to close rather than open.

What worked with Margot was not a clinical explanation. It was a story. Paloma told her about the premonitory urge, not using that term, but describing the experience in physical terms: "Imagine if you had an itch that you physically could not stop scratching, even if you wanted to, even if scratching made people stare. That is what it feels like before a tic. The tic is the scratch." Margot was quiet for a moment. Then she said that sounded exhausting. Paloma said it was. And the conversation they had then was entirely different from every conversation they had attempted before.

The itch-and-scratch metaphor is not original to Paloma. It is one of the most widely used explanatory frameworks in TS communication and one of the most effective because it translates an invisible experience into something almost anyone can feel their way into. Family members who have it available tend to use it again and again, with teachers and employers and strangers, because it works reliably where clinical language does not.

Action challenge: Write a two-minute explanation of TS for someone in your life who does not yet understand it well. Do not use clinical language. Use an analogy, a physical description, or a brief story. Read it aloud. Time it. Trim or expand until it sits comfortably in two minutes. This is the explanation you will use the next time someone needs it.

Summary

The most useful communication in TS families is not the most fluent or the most emotionally generous. It is the most prepared. Silence and brief acknowledgement are often the best response during acute tic episodes, because verbal attention amplifies tic severity. Post-episode conversations work better when they are offered rather than imposed, and when the person with TS chooses when to have them. Treatment conversations work better when they are framed as shared questions rather than proposals. OCD reassurance traps are broken not by refusing to engage but by engaging differently, acknowledging distress without confirming feared content. Extended family conversations work best when clinical language is replaced by physical analogies that translate the invisible experience of TS into something anyone can understand.

Chapter 6 Life Beyond Your Front Door

Clara had been planning her son Martin's twelfth birthday party for three weeks when she realised she was planning it the same way she planned everything: around what would not happen. No crowded indoor venues, because the noise and proximity to strangers amplified his tics and sometimes triggered the vocal sequences she had never learned to name without flinching. No restaurants with open kitchens, because the smells and sounds overlapped in ways that seemed to build pressure in him. No family gatherings larger than eight, because his aunt's reaction the last time had made Martin ask, in the car on the way home, whether he was always going to be embarrassing.

He had asked that question in a flat, factual tone, and Clara had said of course not, and they had both known, in the particular silence that followed, that she had answered the question he asked rather than the one he meant.

The party she planned was small and careful and, in the event, genuinely good. Martin had fun. Nobody stared. Clara spent most of it watching the exits and the faces of other adults and grading each interaction on a scale she had developed over years of attending events with her son. She was exhausted by the time they got home, and Martin fell asleep in the car, and she sat in the driveway for a while before going inside.

The world does not become more hospitable to Tourette Syndrome by being avoided. It becomes more manageable, slowly and imperfectly, through a combination of preparation, practiced responses, and the willingness to re-enter situations that have been difficult rather than simply stop attempting them. This chapter is about that process, and about the family members who carry it alongside the person with TS.

The principle here is direct: public life with TS is not something to be survived through restriction. It is something to be built through preparation, and the family members who prepare best are the ones whose loved ones stay most connected to the world.

Coprolalia Is Rare and Still Changes Everything

Fewer than one in five people with Tourette Syndrome experience coprolalia, the involuntary vocalisation of obscene or socially taboo words and phrases (Zito, 2025). This means that most families reading this chapter will not be navigating coprolalia at all. But for those who are, the experience is so specific and so poorly served by existing resources that it deserves direct treatment here.

Coprolalia is not swearing. This distinction matters enormously and is almost universally misunderstood outside the TS community. Swearing is deliberate, chosen, contextually appropriate or inappropriate based on social judgment. Coprolalia is none of these things. It is a tic, with the same neurological mechanism as any other tic, and the person with TS typically experiences it with the same combination of premonitory urge, brief release, and immediate remorse or embarrassment that characterises all tics. The words produced do not reflect the person's beliefs, intentions, or character. They are, in the most literal clinical sense, involuntary.

The public response to coprolalia does not make this distinction. The public response is usually shock, sometimes anger, and occasionally the kind of sustained attention that creates secondary crisis. For the family members present, the experience is one of secondary stigma: absorbing the reactions directed at someone they love, managing their own visible response, and trying to support the person with TS while the situation resolves.

Marcel, whose wife Ines developed her three-sentence script in the previous chapter, had a coprolalia episode at a supermarket checkout in the second year of their marriage. He did not have coprolalia frequently, but it happened under conditions of elevated anxiety, and waiting in checkout lines was one of those conditions. The word that came out was loud enough for the three customers nearest the checkout to hear. Two of them looked at him. One looked at Ines. Ines had nothing prepared. She said nothing. She put the groceries on the belt and completed the transaction and they walked to the car and she held it together until the car door was closed.

She found a statement, eventually, through a Tourette Association support group. The statement was simple: "My husband has Tourette Syndrome. The word was a tic. He can't control it and it doesn't reflect what he thinks." Twelve words for the stranger who stared. Eighteen for the one who seemed to need more. She put this in her wallet next to the three sentences and did not need it again for eight months, but when she did, it was there.

Prepare Before You Arrive

Pre-event planning is not anxiety management. It is operational preparation, and the distinction matters because anxiety management implies the goal is to feel less anxious, while operational preparation has a different goal: to know what to do before the moment requires knowing it.

The families who navigate public life most effectively with TS are not the least anxious. They are the most prepared. They have thought through the high-risk variables in advance, assigned roles, agreed on exit strategies, and developed a shared vocabulary for the signals that matter. When a situation develops, they do not need to negotiate under pressure. They already know the plan.

A practical pre-event framework has four components. First, the environment assessment: what is the likely tic load in this setting, based on known triggers such as noise, crowds, fluorescent lighting, unpredictable social interactions, and stress? Second, the role assignment: who will handle external communication if needed, and who will focus on the person with TS? Third, the exit strategy: what is the agreed signal for when leaving is the right choice, and how will leaving be managed without escalating the episode? Fourth, the debrief plan: how and when will the family process what happened after the event is over?

This is not a bureaucratic document. For most families, once established, these four questions take about five minutes to run through before any significant public event. The investment is small. The difference it makes in acute moments is considerable.

Coralie and her partner had developed this framework after a wedding where nothing had gone wrong but both of them had been too tense to enjoy themselves because neither knew what they would do if something did go wrong. The next time they attended a wedding, they had fifteen minutes of pre-event planning in the car on the way there. They had a signal, a shared word that meant "I need to step outside," and they had agreed on who would make the social explanation if one was needed. Nothing went wrong that time either, but the evening was entirely different. Coralie danced. Her partner stayed until ten o'clock. They drove home talking about the food.

Action challenge: Before the next public event that carries any significant tic risk, run through the four pre-event questions with the person with TS. Write the answers down if that helps. Agree on the exit signal and the communication role. Notice whether the event itself feels different when the preparation is in place.

Responding to Strangers Without Drama

The stranger who stares, the child who mimics, the adult who confronts, the bystander who offers unwanted commentary: these are the recurring cast of public life with TS, and the family member who has not prepared a response to them will improvise badly in the moment almost every time.

The principle for stranger responses is economy. The more words used, the more explanation offered, the more defensive the tone, the more the incident becomes a scene. A scene extends the duration of the difficult moment and tends to increase tic severity in the person with TS, who is aware of everything happening around them. The goal is not to educate the stranger. The goal is to close the incident with minimum additional stress.

For most situations, a short, neutral statement is more effective than either silence or a full explanation. "He has Tourette Syndrome, it's a tic" is enough in almost every scenario. It answers the question that is being implied, it names the condition without dramatising it, and it returns the situation to ordinary rather than extraordinary. The family member who can say this with the same tone they might use to say the bus is running late has usually ended the situation.

For hostile or persistent strangers, a slightly different tool applies. "I understand you're surprised. He has a neurological condition. We're fine, thank you." The structure here does three things: it acknowledges the stranger's response without agreeing with it, it provides minimal but sufficient information, and it closes with a signal that the exchange is over. The "thank you" is not gratitude. It is punctuation.

Sebastian and Lucia had a version of this they called the "two lines and a turn." Two sentences, and then Sebastian would physically turn to resume whatever he had been doing, which gave Lucia permission to do the same. They had practised it. It had become almost mechanical, and the mechanicalness was the point. Mechanical responses in high-pressure moments are more reliable than creative ones.

After the Hard Day

The debrief after a difficult public episode is a separate conversation from the post-episode conversation described in

Chapter 5. The post-episode conversation is about what happened inside the tic sequence. The debrief after a public event is about what happened around it: what the family member experienced, what the person with TS experienced, what went well, what they would do differently.

This conversation is useful and is often avoided, because it requires both people to be honest about something difficult. The family member may have felt embarrassed, or frightened, or resentful, or proud of themselves for managing well, or guilty for having mixed feelings at all. The person with TS may have felt ashamed, or grateful, or irritated by a response that was well-intentioned but slightly wrong. These are all legitimate responses to a genuinely hard experience, and none of them are well-served by being left unspoken.

The most useful debriefs are specific rather than general. Not "how are you feeling about today" but "the moment when the man at the table next to us said something, what was that like for you?" Not "you seemed upset on the way home" but "I noticed I felt really tense during the checkout. Did you notice that too?" Specific questions produce specific answers, and specific answers are more useful than general reassurances in both directions.

Hugo and Noemi had developed what they called the "three things debrief": one thing that went better than expected, one thing that was harder than expected, and one thing they would do differently. It took twelve minutes in the car on the way home and had become the ritual that made going out worth going.

Action challenge: After the next significant public event, try the three-things debrief format in the car or at home within two hours of returning. Write the three items down together if that helps. Notice whether having a structure for the conversation makes it easier to have than a general check-in.

Building a Life That Goes Somewhere

The families who do best over the long term with TS are not the ones who have the least public difficulty. They are the ones who keep going. They go to the events, and some events go badly, and they go again. They build a repertoire of environments that are reliably manageable, and they add new ones cautiously, and they return to the ones that were difficult until they are no longer difficult. The world does not expand by being observed from the inside.

This matters because the alternative, the slow contraction of social life around the avoidances that feel safe, has a long-term cost that is easy to miss year by year and unmistakable decade by decade. Julian and Mateo's grocery shopping story in Chapter 4 is the small version of this story. The large version is a family that has stopped going to weddings, stopped visiting relatives, stopped eating at restaurants, stopped taking holidays, stopped inviting anyone over, and has arrived at a life that is technically undisruptive and entirely diminished.

The goal is not to eliminate tic episodes from public life. That is not achievable and is not the right target. The goal is to build a family life that is full enough, connected enough, and enjoyable enough that the episodes that happen in the middle of it are incidents rather than catastrophes.

Clara's son is fourteen now. He went to a birthday party last month at a crowded bowling alley, the kind of environment Clara spent years avoiding on his behalf. He ticced throughout. He came home at eleven o'clock, tired and happy, and told her the birthday cake had been excellent. Clara stood in the kitchen for a moment after he went upstairs, not because something had been achieved but because something had been preserved.

Summary

Coprolalia affects fewer than one in five people with TS, but for those families it does affect, preparation and practiced responses make an enormous difference in how incidents are managed and recovered from. Pre-event planning, running through environment, roles, exits, and debrief before significant public events, reduces in-the-moment pressure and produces better outcomes. Stranger responses work best when they are short, neutral, and rehearsed rather than improvised under stress. The post-event debrief is a separate and important conversation from the post-episode conversation, and specific questions produce more useful exchanges than general check-ins. The families whose loved ones stay most connected to the world are the ones who keep going despite the episodes, not the ones who succeed in avoiding them.

Chapter 7 Advocate Without Apology

Eloise had been to four meetings at her daughter's school before she understood that she had been attending them wrong.

Not wrong in preparation. She had prepared. She had brought printed articles about Tourette Syndrome, a list of her daughter's specific tic patterns, and a set of notes organised under headings that she had typed the evening before. She had been thorough, accurate, and, in the memory of every meeting, fairly easy to dismiss. The special educational needs coordinator had thanked her for the materials and promised to share them with the classroom teachers. The head of year had expressed sympathy and mentioned that several of the teachers were already very supportive. The SENCO at the next school year had asked whether the tics were perhaps related to anxiety at home and suggested the school counsellor as a resource.

None of these meetings had produced anything that changed what happened to her daughter during the school day.

The fifth meeting was different. Eloise arrived without the printed articles. She had spent the day before writing a single page, clearly titled "What my daughter needs to succeed in your school," which contained three numbered items with the specific support she was requesting and the specific reason for each. She had not framed these as requests. She had framed them as provisions, because her daughter was entitled to them under the law. She had not been apologetic. She had been specific, calm, and ready to stay in the room until the items were agreed.

The meeting lasted forty-five minutes. Three provisions were agreed in writing. Eloise's daughter got a seat at the end of the row, permission to leave class briefly when tic pressure became unmanageable, and a brief standardised explanation given to her class by a school nurse rather than by the teacher who had, twice, handled tic episodes in ways that caused her to cry in the car on the way home.

The difference between the first four meetings and the fifth was not Eloise's knowledge. It was her positioning. She had stopped attending as a parent who was hoping for goodwill and started attending as a person who understood what her child was entitled to receive.

The principle of this chapter is that advocacy for a family member with TS is most effective not when it is most sympathetic but when it is most specific. Sympathy invites discretion. Specificity invites action. The family members who get results for the people they love are the ones who come in with exact language, legal grounding, and a clear understanding that they are not asking for a favour.

What Schools Are Required to Provide

In the United States, students with Tourette Syndrome may be eligible for accommodations under two frameworks: a Section 504 plan or an Individualized Education Program. Understanding the difference between these determines the correct strategy for any given meeting.

A Section 504 plan, under the Rehabilitation Act of 1973, applies to students whose disability substantially limits a major life activity, which for TS typically includes learning, concentrating, and communicating. Section 504 does not require the student to need special education services; it requires only that the school provide equal access through reasonable accommodations. Common TS-relevant 504 accommodations include extended time on assessments, preferential seating, permission for brief breaks, reduced or modified homework when tic-related fatigue is a factor, and a private room for high-stakes testing.

An Individualized Education Program, available under the Individuals with Disabilities Education Act, applies when the disability adversely affects educational performance to the degree that the student needs specially designed instruction. Students whose TS-Plus profile includes significant ADHD, learning disabilities, or anxiety that impairs academic function may qualify for an IEP rather than, or in addition to, a 504 plan.

In the United Kingdom, the equivalent framework is an Education, Health and Care plan under the Children and Families Act 2014. The EHC plan is available when a student's needs cannot be met through standard school-based support, and it carries legal force once issued. Parents in England have rights to request an EHC assessment at any point, and local authorities are legally required to respond within six weeks.

In Australia, the Nationally Consistent Collection of Data framework identifies students with disability and determines the adjustments schools are required to provide under the Disability Standards for Education 2005. Schools are legally required to make reasonable adjustments for students with TS, and parents have the right to participate in the development of those adjustments.

Knowing which framework applies is the first step. The second is arriving at the meeting with specific accommodations already named, rather than a general request for support, because general requests produce general responses and general responses are easy to deprioritise.

Action challenge: Find out which framework applies to the student with TS in your family, based on your country and your school district. Write down the three specific accommodations that would make the most difference to their daily experience. Frame them as entitlements, not requests. Bring this list to your next school meeting.

Language That Opens Doors

The language used in school and workplace advocacy is not incidental to the outcome. It is a significant determinant of it. Certain formulations invite resistance. Others close it down before it starts.

Formulations that invite resistance: "I was wondering if it might be possible for the school to consider..." and "I know you are all very busy, but perhaps if there were any opportunity to..." and "I don't want to be a difficult parent, but..." These formulations signal that the speaker expects pushback and is pre-apologising for taking up space. They set up a negotiation where the other party holds most of the advantage.

Formulations that produce results: "I am writing to confirm our agreement that..." and "Under Section 504, my child is entitled to..." and "I would like these accommodations documented in writing before the next assessment." These formulations are not aggressive. They are precise. They treat the meeting as what it actually is: a formal process with specific obligations attached, not a conversation about goodwill.

Zoe, a parent of two children in the same school district, had found a single sentence that she used to open every accommodation meeting: "I am here today because my child has a documented neurological condition, and I want to make sure we leave this meeting with a written plan that supports their education. I am happy to discuss the details of that plan now." She reported that the tone of meetings changed immediately after she began using this sentence, and that the written plans she received after it were more specific and more durable than the ones she had received before.

The difference is not confrontational framing. It is competent framing, and there is a meaningful distinction between the two.

Workplace Disclosure for Adults with TS

The adult with TS navigating workplace disclosure faces a different set of calculations from the school-age child, and the family member who is supporting that process needs to understand what is at stake in those calculations.

In the United States, the Americans with Disabilities Act requires employers with 15 or more employees to provide reasonable accommodations for employees with documented disabilities, including Tourette Syndrome. The employee is not required to disclose the specific diagnosis; they are required only to request an accommodation and indicate that it is related to a medical condition. The employer may ask for documentation from a healthcare provider but may not ask for details of the diagnosis itself.

In the United Kingdom, the Equality Act 2010 provides similar protection. Tourette Syndrome meets the legal definition of a disability under the Act if it has a substantial and long-term adverse effect on the ability to carry out normal day-to-day activities. Employers are required to make reasonable adjustments, which for TS typically include modified seating arrangements, reduced noise environments, flexible working arrangements where tics make standard commute or schedule demands unmanageable, and understanding around intermittent absences related to tic severity or medical appointments.

The practical question for most adults with TS is not whether to disclose but when and to whom. Research on workplace disclosure in neurological and psychiatric conditions consistently finds that selective disclosure, to a direct line manager or HR contact rather than to the wider workplace, produces better outcomes than full disclosure or complete non-disclosure (Corrigan et al., 2016). The family member's role in this process is to provide information and support for the decision, not to drive it.

Felix disclosed his TS to his manager in the third year of his current job, after a tic episode in a client meeting created an awkward situation that he had been unable to contextualise in the moment. He prepared a brief written statement, one paragraph, that named the condition, described its primary manifestations in his work context, requested one specific accommodation, and indicated his willingness to answer questions. His manager read it, asked two questions, and agreed to the accommodation in an email that afternoon. Felix said later that the preparation had taken longer than the conversation.

When Institutions Do Not Comply

Some schools and some employers do not respond well to accommodation requests, regardless of how those requests are framed. When this happens, the family member needs to know the escalation pathway and be willing to use it.

In the United States, complaints about school non-compliance under Section 504 are filed with the Office for Civil Rights at the Department of Education. IDEA non-compliance complaints go to the relevant state education agency. Both processes are free and do not require a lawyer at the initial stage, though legal support becomes useful if the complaint proceeds.

In the United Kingdom, disputes about EHC plans are resolved through the SEND Tribunal, which is a free service available to parents and young people in England. The Tourette Association UK provides guidance on this process and can refer families to advocacy organisations.

The willingness to escalate is sometimes all that is needed. Schools and employers who have been non-compliant tend to become responsive when they understand that the family member knows the escalation process and is prepared to use it. This is not a threat. It is information about where the conversation goes if the current approach does not produce results.

Eloise has never needed to escalate. But she knows the exact steps for doing so, and she mentioned them in passing at the fifth meeting, not as a threat, as a matter of professional knowledge. Nobody at that meeting tested her.

Accommodating TS-Plus, Not Just TS

The final and often overlooked element of school and workplace advocacy is the distinction between accommodating TS itself and accommodating the full TS-Plus profile. An accommodation plan that addresses tics but not ADHD-related executive function difficulties, or that allows for breaks but does not address OCD-driven delays, is a partial plan.

As discussed in Chapter 2, the majority of people with TS also have ADHD, OCD, anxiety, or some combination of these. Each of these conditions has its own accommodation implications. ADHD warrants chunked task presentation, frequent check-ins, movement breaks, and reduced demand for sustained attention without breaks. OCD-related rituals and "not just right" experiences may require extensions and a private space. Anxiety warrants advance notice of schedule changes, reduced performance pressure in front of peers, and access to a trusted adult when tic severity is elevated.

An accommodation plan that addresses all of these, mapped to the individual student's or employee's specific profile, is substantially more useful than one that names Tourette Syndrome and stops there.

The family member's role in building this plan is to bring the full TS-Plus picture to the meeting, named specifically and documented where possible. A one-page summary from the treating clinician, confirming the diagnoses and their educational or occupational implications, is a more effective document in these meetings than the most carefully printed academic article.

Action challenge: If a school or workplace accommodation plan exists for the person with TS in your family, review it this week. List every condition in the TS-Plus profile. Check whether each condition is addressed in the plan. Note the gaps. Bring a specific addition for each gap to the next review meeting.

Summary

Accommodation advocacy works best when it is specific, legally grounded, and framed as entitlement rather than request. In the United States, Section 504 and IEP frameworks provide legal obligations for school accommodations; in the UK, EHC plans provide equivalent force; in Australia, the Disability Standards for Education apply. Workplace disclosure in adults with TS works best when it is selective, prepared, and accompanied by a specific written accommodation request. When institutions fail to comply, escalation pathways are free, clearly defined, and often need only to be named. And the most complete accommodation plans address the full TS-Plus profile rather than tics alone.

Chapter 8 Know Your Treatment Options

Valeria had a spreadsheet. It had four columns: the date, the medication, the dose, and a brief note about what happened. The spreadsheet covered three years and nine different medication trials. Some of the notes were clinical, things like "reduced tic frequency approximately 30%, significant fatigue" and "no measurable effect, discontinued at week six." Some of the notes were not clinical. One said: "Felix cried on the phone from work. Said he could not feel his hands right."

She had built the spreadsheet because, by the third year, she could not remember which medication had caused which problem. The things that had been tried blurred into each other, separated only by the notes she had started keeping after the second trial, when it occurred to her that nobody else was tracking the full picture. The neurologist had the prescribing record. The GP had a summary letter. Felix had the experience. Valeria had the spreadsheet, which was to say that Valeria had the clearest view of the three years.

The referral to a CBIT therapist happened in the thirty-seventh month. The neurologist mentioned it, almost in passing, after a review appointment at which Valeria had brought the spreadsheet and spread it on the desk and pointed to the pattern visible in columns three and four. The neurologist looked at the spreadsheet for a long moment and then said that he thought it might be time to try a different approach. He wrote the referral while they were still in the room.

The CBIT therapist they found saw Felix for twelve weeks. By week eight, the tics that had been most disruptive to his working life had reduced by more than half. By week twelve, he was using a competing response in meetings without anyone noticing he was doing anything at all. The spreadsheet's final entry, written by Valeria six months after the last appointment, said: "Better. Actually better."

She had not known what CBIT was at the start of the three years. Felix had not known. The neurologist had not mentioned it until month thirty-seven. The family had spent three years in a treatment process that was not organised around the best available evidence, and they had done so not from carelessness but from a simple absence of information.

This chapter provides the information. The treatment landscape for Tourette Syndrome is better than most families encounter in their early years, and understanding it is the beginning of making better decisions.

The principle is this: the most effective TS treatment available is not medication. It is a specific form of behavioural therapy, and most families have not been told this. Knowing the evidence hierarchy, and knowing how to advocate for movement within it, is one of the most practically useful things a family member can do.

CBIT Is First-Line Treatment

Comprehensive Behavioral Intervention for Tics, known as CBIT and pronounced "see-bit," is the treatment that the American Academy of Neurology names as the recommended first-line approach for Tourette Syndrome and persistent tic disorders (Pringsheim et al., 2019). It is also the treatment that most families do not hear about until they have already been through a medication trial or several.

CBIT is not relaxation therapy. It is not a version of telling someone to calm down. It is a structured, manualised treatment built on the neurological reality of the premonitory urge. Its core mechanism, habit reversal training, teaches the person with TS to recognise the premonitory urge as it builds and to perform a competing movement or behaviour that is physically incompatible with the tic. The competing response reduces or prevents the tic without suppressing it in the way that voluntary suppression does, because it works with the urge rather than against it.

Large-scale, NIH-funded clinical trials have found that more than half of people who complete CBIT show significant reductions in tic severity, and that these reductions are maintained at six-month follow-up (Piacentini et al., 2010; Wilhelm et al., 2012). A direct comparison with antipsychotic medication found CBIT to be as effective as medication in reducing tics, with a more favourable side-effect profile (Pringsheim et al., 2019). These are not preliminary findings. They are the evidence base on which the AAN treatment guidelines are built.

For family members, the practical implication is that if CBIT has not been recommended or offered, it is worth asking for it directly. A referral to a CBIT-trained therapist is a reasonable first-line request at any neurology or psychiatry appointment, regardless of how long medication-based treatment has been in progress.

How to find a CBIT therapist: the Tourette Association of America maintains a provider directory at tourette.org. The Tourette Action UK has a similar resource. Therapists with CBIT training will typically list this credential explicitly. If no CBIT-trained therapist is available in the local area, telehealth delivery of CBIT has been studied and found effective (Ricketts et al., 2016).

The Family's Role in CBIT

CBIT is not something that happens to the person with TS while the family member waits outside. For children and adolescents, family involvement is built into the treatment protocol. For adults, the family member's role is less formalised but no less important.

The family component of CBIT, particularly for children, includes psychoeducation about tics and the premonitory urge, training in how to respond to tics during treatment, and guidance on how to modify daily routines in ways that support treatment goals (Woods et al., 2007). This last element draws directly on the principles of Chapter 4: the family member's behaviour in the home environment is a variable in the treatment outcome.

Specifically, CBIT asks family members to stop providing attention to tics during the treatment period, which reinforces the neutral-responding approach discussed earlier. It also asks family members to support practice of competing responses at home, which means knowing what the competing response is and providing a supportive environment for practising it without turning practice into performance pressure. And it asks family members to be aware of the functional assessment findings, which identify specific situations that reliably precede or worsen tic episodes, so that the home environment can be modified where possible.

Noemi, who had worked through the CBIT process with Hugo, described her role as something like a spotter at a gym: not doing the exercise, not coaching the form, just present in a way that made it safer to try things. She said this was harder than it sounded, because she was an organised person who liked to help efficiently, and efficient helpful people in CBIT settings sometimes make the treatment harder rather than easier. She had learned to hold back, and the holding back had been its own kind of contribution.

Action challenge: If CBIT is currently in progress or being considered, ask the CBIT therapist directly what your role in the treatment should be. Write down the answer. Make one specific change to your home behaviour that aligns with what the therapist describes. Track whether that change correlates with any difference in tic frequency or episode intensity over two weeks.

Medication in Plain Language

Medication for Tourette Syndrome is not a failure and is not a last resort. For many people with TS, particularly those whose tic severity is high enough to cause physical injury, significant social impairment, or educational failure, medication is a reasonable and sometimes necessary component of treatment. The evidence base for several medication classes is solid. The question for most families is not whether medication is legitimate but which medication, when, and why.

The alpha-agonist medications, guanfacine and clonidine, are typically the first medications trialled for tics in children. They are not specifically tic medications; they were developed for blood pressure and attention, but they have documented efficacy in reducing tic severity, and their side-effect profile is more acceptable than the alternatives for most families. Clonidine in particular can also assist with the sleep difficulties discussed in Chapter 2, which makes it useful for the TS-Plus profile where both tics and sleep disruption are present (Tourette Syndrome Study Group, 2002).

Antipsychotic medications, including aripiprazole, haloperidol, pimozide, and risperidone, have the strongest evidence base for tic reduction but also carry more significant side-effect risks, including weight gain, metabolic changes, and in some cases movement side effects that can be difficult to distinguish from the tics being treated. They are typically considered after alpha-agonists have been tried or when tic severity is high enough to warrant a stronger intervention.

Topiramate, an anticonvulsant, has been studied for tic reduction and shows moderate efficacy with a different side-effect profile from antipsychotics, including cognitive slowing at higher doses (Jankovic et al., 2010). It is sometimes used when antipsychotics are not tolerated.

For TS-Plus profiles where OCD is significantly impairing, selective serotonin reuptake inhibitors are the standard pharmacological treatment, but they are not tic medications. They address the OCD component specifically and should be understood as a separate treatment target from the tics.

The medication conversation with a neurologist or psychiatrist is more productive when the family member has a clear account of what has been tried, what effect it had, and what the current priorities are. Valeria's spreadsheet is an extreme example, but its underlying principle is sound: the person who has tracked the full picture has a more useful conversation with the prescribing clinician than the person who is reconstructing it from memory.

Deep Brain Stimulation and When It Applies

Deep brain stimulation, or DBS, is a surgical intervention in which electrodes are implanted in specific brain regions and connected to a device that delivers continuous electrical stimulation. For Tourette Syndrome, DBS is considered only in cases of severe, treatment-refractory tics that have not responded to multiple adequate trials of medication and behavioural therapy and that are causing significant injury or profound functional impairment.

DBS is not a common treatment for TS, and families who are not facing severe refractory cases do not need to be actively considering it. What is worth knowing is that it is available as a specialist intervention, that outcomes in carefully selected adult patients have been promising in multiple case series and small controlled studies, and that evaluation for DBS appropriateness happens at specialist movement disorder centres rather than general neurology practices (Baldermann et al., 2016).

For the small number of families for whom DBS is a genuine consideration, the first step is a referral from a movement disorder neurologist to a centre with specific TS-DBS experience. The evaluation process is lengthy and involves multidisciplinary assessment. This is appropriate: DBS is an irreversible surgical intervention and the evaluation standards reflect that.

Supporting Treatment at Home

The family member's most consistent contribution to any treatment approach, behavioural or pharmacological, is the home environment they create. This means the neutral responding discussed in Chapter 4, the pre-event planning from Chapter 6, the communication approaches from Chapter 5, and the specific CBIT support discussed earlier in this chapter. It also means something simpler: showing up to appointments, keeping records, noticing what changes, and raising what is not working with thc clinical team rather than absorbing it silently.

Marcel's treatment history before he found an effective combination involved two failed medication trials and one CBIT course that ended prematurely because his therapist relocated. What made the third attempt different was that Ines had been to the previous appointments and had notes. When they met the new neurologist, Ines pulled out a brief written summary, one page, covering what had been tried, what had worked partially, what had caused problems, and what Marcel's current priorities were. The neurologist said, near the end of the appointment, that this was the most useful first appointment she had ever had with a new patient.

Ines had written the summary in forty minutes. Marcel had reviewed it and said it was accurate. It had taken less effort than many of the things they had done in those years that had not helped. The simplest tools are often the ones that get overlooked.

Action challenge: Write a one-page treatment summary for the person with TS in your life. Include the treatments that have been tried, the effect of each, any side effects or problems, and the current treatment goals. Keep it factual. Bring it to the next clinical appointment. Notice whether it changes the quality of the conversation.

Summary

CBIT is the AAN-recommended first-line treatment for Tourette Syndrome and should be the starting point of any serious treatment conversation, regardless of how long medication-based approaches have been underway. The family member's role in CBIT is active and specific: neutral responding, home practice support, and environment modification based on the functional assessment. Medication is a legitimate and sometimes necessary treatment component, and the alpha-agonists are typically the first pharmacological approach for children. Antipsychotics have the strongest evidence base for tic reduction but carry more significant side-effect risks. DBS is available for severe refractory cases in specialist centres. The family member's most consistent contribution to any treatment process is the quality of information they bring to clinical appointments and the home environment they create between them.

Chapter 9 Build a Home That Helps

For two years, Zoe answered the same question forty times a day.

The question changed in form but not in substance. Was the stove off. Had she locked the front door. Was Gabriel going to be safe at school. Was she sure. Was she completely sure. The question had a slightly different texture each time, a slight variation in what certainty was being requested, and Zoe, who was a careful and attentive parent, worked hard to provide the exact answer that each variation required. She did this because providing the answer made Gabriel calm, briefly. And because she could not watch her son be distressed and do nothing.

At the height of this period, she was spending between forty-five minutes and an hour each morning answering questions before Gabriel could get out the door. She had stopped noticing how long it took. She had stopped noticing how often the same question returned, and how the return always came faster than the last time, and how the reassurance she provided never seemed to be quite enough to last more than a few minutes. She noticed only that mornings were hard, that Gabriel was suffering, and that answering the questions was the one thing she could do that made any visible difference.

She found out that she had been making things worse from a therapist who specialised in OCD. The therapist explained, in a quiet and non-accusatory way, that Gabriel's OCD was functioning like a lock that required a key. Reassurance was the key. Every time Zoe provided the key, the lock came back. The reason Gabriel needed reassurance more frequently over time was not that his OCD was getting worse in some external sense. It was that Zoe had been reliably providing the mechanism that OCD needed to sustain itself.

Zoe sat in the car after that appointment for a long time.

She did not blame herself, ultimately. She had done what any parent would do. She had looked at a child in distress and responded to the distress with whatever worked in the moment. The problem was that the thing that worked in the moment was also the thing that made the moment more likely to return. Nobody had explained this to her before. Nobody had told her that the home environment she created was a clinical variable in her child's OCD, not a background setting but an active participant.

That appointment changed how Zoe ran her household. Not dramatically, not overnight, and not without difficulty. But it changed. And over the following eight months, the forty daily reassurances became twenty, then ten, then a handful. The mornings became usable again. Gabriel still had OCD. He also learned, slowly, that he could tolerate the uncertainty without the key.

The home environment is not a neutral container for TS-Plus. It is an active ingredient in how well or poorly the TS-Plus profile is managed on any given day. The principle of this chapter is this: the family member who understands how the home environment interacts with OCD, ADHD, rage attacks, and sleep disruption can make changes that produce measurable improvements, without medication, without therapy, and without waiting for a specialist appointment.

Reassurance Makes OCD Worse

The reassurance trap, introduced in Chapter 5 as a communication problem, is also a household structure problem. When a household is organised around the provision of OCD reassurance, including shared rituals, avoided objects or topics, or the family member's involvement in checking behaviours, the OCD is being maintained by the home environment as much as by the person with TS.

Research on family accommodation in OCD, the term clinicians use for the ways family members adjust their behaviour to manage OCD symptoms, consistently finds that higher accommodation is associated with greater OCD severity and poorer treatment outcomes (Storch et al., 2007). The family members who accommodate most are often the most caring. The accommodation is an expression of love. It is also, in clinical terms, a maintaining factor.

The corrective is gradual rather than sudden. Cutting off all reassurance immediately tends to produce a distress spike that the family member cannot sustain, which leads to resuming the accommodation and increasing the OCD's confidence that persistence pays. A graduated approach, working ideally with a therapist trained in exposure and response prevention, involves identifying the most costly accommodations and reducing them incrementally, starting with the ones that are slightly easier to change rather than the most entrenched.

For families without immediate access to a specialist, the first step is simpler: stop adding new accommodations. Before making any major household change, ask whether the change is being made to support the person with TS or to manage the OCD. Buying a lock for the stove because the person with TS finds it uncomfortable when they cannot verify it is off is an accommodation that may relieve distress today and increase OCD severity over the following month. Rearranging the kitchen to reduce a genuine safety hazard is a different kind of change. The distinction matters.

Action challenge: List every accommodation your household currently makes for OCD-related behaviours in the person with TS. Include repeated questions you answer, items you have removed or avoided, things you check on their behalf, and rituals you participate in. Do not judge the list. Count the items. Choose the one that you assess as easiest to modify, and discuss with the person with TS or a treating therapist what a small, gradual reduction might look like.

Structure Reduces ADHD's Impact

ADHD in the context of TS is the condition that most consistently rewards household investment. Unlike OCD, where the family member's best response to the symptom is often restraint, ADHD responds well to the active creation of external structure that substitutes for the internal regulatory capacity the person with TS has in reduced supply.

Hugo's partner Noemi discovered this through a process of accidental experimentation. She had started keeping a whiteboard in their kitchen during a period when she was managing several overlapping work projects and needed to track her own tasks visually. Hugo, who had never asked for any particular household accommodation and who described himself as someone who preferred to keep things in his head, started using the whiteboard too. Not deliberately. He simply began gravitating toward it in the mornings, writing his own tasks alongside hers, checking items off in the afternoon. His appointment-keeping improved. His forgetfulness about household tasks reduced. Neither of them had planned this.

What Noemi had accidentally created was an external executive function system, a physical structure that reduced the demand on Hugo's working memory and attention. The whiteboard was doing what his prefrontal cortex found difficult to do reliably: holding information still and making it visible.

Research on ADHD consistently identifies external organisation systems as among the most effective non-pharmacological supports for executive function difficulties (Barkley, 2006). These systems work not because they change the underlying neurology but because they reduce the cognitive load the neurology is asked to carry. The person with ADHD still has reduced executive function. The external system compensates for the deficit rather than demanding that the person overcome it through effort.

For households with TS-Plus and significant ADHD, the most useful external systems typically address three domains: task management, time management, and environment management. Task management means making tasks visible, in writing, on a surface the person with TS will actually encounter rather than in a phone they do not check. Time management means building in transitions and warnings rather than expecting the person with TS to track elapsed time internally. Environment management means reducing the number of decisions the environment requires, through predictable storage locations, consistent routines, and the elimination of clutter that creates both distraction and demand.

None of these changes require the person with TS to become more organised. They require the household to be organised in ways that reduce the gap between what the person with TS can do and what the household requires of them.

Action challenge: Identify the three ADHD-related household frictions that most consistently cause conflict or difficulty in your home. For each one, design one specific environmental change that reduces the demand rather than asking the person with TS to manage it through effort. Implement one of the three changes this week. Notice over two weeks whether the friction that change addressed has reduced.

Rage Attacks Need a Plan Before They Happen

The rage attack, as described in Chapter 2, is neurologically driven and typically fast: rapid onset, intense peak, quick resolution, genuine remorse. The family member who has not prepared a response to rage attacks before they happen is in the worst possible position when one occurs. The family member who has prepared, who has discussed what is needed and what helps, and who has a shared agreement with the person with TS about what the attack requires, is in a fundamentally different position.

The preparation conversation is one of the most important conversations a TS family can have, and it must happen at a calm, low-stakes moment rather than in the aftermath of an attack when everyone is still recovering. The conversation has three parts. First, what does the person with TS need during a rage attack? For most people, the answer includes reduced verbal interaction, physical space, and the absence of additional demands. Second, what does the family member need in order to provide that? This may include a brief withdrawal from the room, a signal that the attack is over, or a plan for the repair conversation that comes later. Third, what does the safety plan look like for the rare case where the intensity of the attack creates physical risk? This last question is not alarmist. It is responsible.

Oscar had his first preparation conversation with his partner when their therapist suggested it, about fourteen months into their relationship. He had been resistant to the idea, partly because the conversation required him to look directly at something he preferred to manage by not looking at it. He described the rage attacks to his partner, in that conversation, as events that felt entirely alien to him, as though they were happening to someone else while he watched from a distance. He said that the worst part was not the attack itself but the look on her face during it. His partner said that the worst part for her was not knowing what to do. They agreed on a signal, a specific phrase he would say when he felt the pressure building, and on what she would do when she heard it.

They used the signal for the first time six weeks later. The attack did not happen. The signal had given him enough external anchor to redirect the building pressure, which neither of them had anticipated but both of them were glad for.

Safety planning is not a prediction of violence. It is an acknowledgement that some moments require a plan that is already agreed, because in the moment, agreement is not possible.

Sleep Is a System, Not an Event

The sleep difficulties associated with TS-Plus are not random. They follow patterns that, once identified, can be addressed with specific household changes that reduce the overall tic and anxiety load the following day.

As noted in Chapter 2, sleep disruption in TS is linked to several overlapping factors: tics that continue into lighter sleep stages, anxiety that makes falling asleep difficult, and the delayed sleep phase that frequently accompanies ADHD (Ghosh et al., 2014). Each of these has different household implications, and addressing them together produces better results than addressing them individually.

For tics during sleep, the most consistently reported household adjustment is the sleep environment itself. Darkness, lower temperatures, and reduced sensory stimulation are associated with improved sleep quality across the general population and appear particularly relevant for people with TS, whose nervous systems are already managing elevated baseline arousal. Partners who share a bed with someone with TS often find that separate sleep arrangements during high-tic periods, presented as a practical rather than relational choice, reduce sleep disruption for both people without changing the quality of the relationship.

For anxiety-driven insomnia, the household variable with the most consistent support is the wind-down period. Research on sleep and anxiety consistently finds that the hour before bed functions as preparation rather than transition: the activities that happen in it prime the nervous system for either rest or continued activation (Harvey, 2002). Screens that carry social or work content, conversations about difficult topics, and environments that remain stimulating until the moment of attempted sleep all prime for activation. Quiet, dim, low-demand activity in the hour before bed primes in the other direction.

Mateo and Julian restructured their evenings after a sustained period in which Mateo's sleep was poor enough to affect his daytime tic severity, his emotional regulation, and his capacity to manage the executive demands of his work. The restructuring was specific. The phone screen was removed from the bedroom. The evening's final hour became predictable and low-stimulation. Julian took over the tasks that had been happening in that hour, so that Mateo's last activity before sleep was not catching up on anything but something more neutral. The improvement was visible within ten days. It was not a cure. It was a system adjustment that changed the baseline.

Action challenge: Run a low-demand household audit this week. Walk through a typical day from the perspective of the person with TS and note every point where the environment makes an unnecessary demand on executive function, attention, sensory tolerance, or OCD management. Write down five specific changes you could make to the home environment that would reduce the total daily demand. Choose one and implement it before the next week is out.

When to Bring in Additional Support

There are conditions in the TS-Plus profile that respond well to professional support beyond the standard neurologist and psychiatrist. Knowing who those professionals are and when to involve them is a practical piece of knowledge that most families do not have until they stumble upon it.

Occupational therapists with neurodevelopmental experience are particularly useful for sensory processing difficulties that co-occur with TS-Plus, for fine motor difficulties that sometimes accompany the condition, and for building daily living structures that reduce the executive function demand of household routines. An OT who understands ADHD can reframe an entire kitchen in two appointments.

Educational psychologists provide assessments that identify specific learning profiles in students with TS-Plus, assessments that are frequently required for school accommodation applications and that can reveal learning difficulties that were previously attributed to laziness or attitude. The assessment that Hugo received, discussed in Chapter 2, is the educational psychology model applied to an adult. For children, this assessment is often the document that unlocks the school support described in Chapter 7.

ADHD coaches, working as a complement to medical treatment rather than a replacement for it, provide the practical support structures that medication alone does not. They help the person with TS build external systems, routines, and accountability structures that compensate for executive function deficits in daily life. They also work with family members on how to support structure-building without becoming the structure, which is the central challenge for every partner and parent in a TS-Plus household.

Clara, whose son Martin had TS, ADHD, and anxiety, brought in an OT in Martin's seventh year after a school report described his handwriting and fine motor performance as significantly below his academic ability. The OT found sensory processing differences that had never been flagged, made two specific environmental modifications to Martin's homework space, and recommended a particular pen grip that reduced the physical effort of writing enough that Martin completed his homework with less protest within three weeks. The OT had seen Martin for four sessions. Clara had been fighting about homework for two years.

Summary

The home environment is not a passive setting for TS-Plus. It is an active participant in how well the TS-Plus profile is managed each day. Providing OCD reassurance maintains the OCD and must be reduced gradually, ideally with professional support. ADHD responds well to external structure that reduces executive function demand rather than demanding that the person with TS manage it through effort alone. Rage attacks need a preparation conversation at a calm moment, with agreed signals, agreed responses, and a safety plan for the rare event of elevated intensity. Sleep disruption follows identifiable patterns, and specific household changes to the sleep environment and the wind-down period produce measurable improvements. Occupational therapists, educational psychologists, and ADHD coaches provide specialist support that most families discover too late.

Chapter 10 When Tics Come Out of Nowhere

Lucia's son Elio was nine years old and, by every observable measure, thriving. He was doing well at school, sleeping without difficulty, playing with friends on weekends, and showing no sign of any of the conditions that ran in both sides of the family. Lucia had noticed a habit of eye-blinking that seemed to come and go, which she had mentioned to the paediatrician at the previous year's check-up. The paediatrician had said to keep an eye on it.

She was not worried about Elio. This is the detail that stayed with her later, that she had not been worried, that she had gone to bed on a Tuesday night with an ordinary sense of ordinary family life proceeding in an ordinary direction.

On Wednesday morning, Elio could not stop washing his hands. He had to wash them until they felt right, and they did not feel right for a very long time. He was also afraid, suddenly and intensely, in ways he had not been afraid before: of dogs, of the dark, of something unspecified but persistent that he could not name and that made him clutch her arm in public spaces they had walked through a hundred times without incident. He was also making sounds. A rapid, low, repeated vocalisation that he could not explain and did not seem to notice he was making.

Within forty-eight hours, Lucia had a son who seemed to be a different child. He said to her, on Thursday evening, in a voice that was frightened in a way nine-year-olds rarely allow themselves to be: "I don't know what's wrong with me."

She did not know either. She had no language for what had happened and no framework for understanding it. The paediatrician, when she called the next morning, used words she had to look up. The immunologist she saw three weeks later, after significant difficulty getting a referral, used different words. The specialist she finally reached, six months into what she would later describe as the worst period of her adult life, used the word PANDAS, and when she looked it up that evening she sat in the bathroom with her phone for a long time because the description matched her son so precisely that it felt like reading a document that had been written about him specifically.

The principle of this chapter is simple and important: sudden, dramatic onset of tics, OCD, anxiety, or behavioural change in a child without a prior TS history is not the same clinical picture as gradual-onset Tourette Syndrome. It is a specific and identifiable pattern that has a name, a research base, and a treatment pathway. The families who find that pathway fastest are the ones who knew what to look for.

Understand the Difference From Classic TS

Tourette Syndrome develops gradually. Tics typically begin between the ages of five and seven, with motor tics appearing before vocal tics, and with the full TS picture establishing itself over months to years (Robertson et al., 2017). The onset is not dramatic. Parents often describe not being able to identify a clear starting point, only a retrospective sense that the tics were there for a while before they were noticed.

PANS and PANDAS are entirely different in their onset. PANDAS stands for pediatric autoimmune neuropsychiatric disorders associated with streptococcal infections. PANS stands for pediatric acute-onset neuropsychiatric syndrome. In both conditions, the onset is sudden, often occurring within 24 to 48 hours of an infection or other immune system activation. Parents describe the change as happening overnight. They use phrases like "he woke up a different child" and "she just suddenly wasn't herself." The speed and severity of the change is the feature that most clearly distinguishes PANS and PANDAS from classic TS.

The primary symptom in PANS and PANDAS is severe OCD, often accompanied by tics, extreme anxiety, dramatic mood and behavioural changes, regression in previously mastered skills, sleep disruption, and physical symptoms including urinary frequency and fine motor deterioration (Chang et al., 2015). Children with PANDAS have a documented history of streptococcal infection preceding the acute episode. Children with PANS have a broader range of possible immune triggers, including other infections and inflammatory events.

Children with PANS and PANDAS may receive a TS diagnosis if the tic component is prominent, but they represent a clinically distinct population. Research estimates that PANS and PANDAS may account for as many as 25 percent of children diagnosed with OCD and tic disorders (Snider & Swedo, 2004). This is not a rare phenomenon affecting a handful of families.

Recognise the Signs Early

The single most important thing a family member can do when dramatic and sudden behavioural change occurs in a child is to document it precisely. The day it started. What the child was doing the week before. Whether there was any illness, any fever, any sore throat, any unusual fatigue in the month preceding the onset. Whether the symptoms appeared over hours or days. What the specific symptoms are.

This documentation matters because the diagnosis of PANS and PANDAS is clinical. There is no single definitive laboratory test. The specialist who evaluates the child is making a judgment based on the history, the symptom pattern, and the laboratory findings together. A parent who can provide a precise and detailed history is contributing materially to the accuracy of that judgment. A parent who is reconstructing events from weeks-old memory is at a disadvantage, as is the child.

The diagnostic criteria for PANS, as established by research guidelines, require sudden dramatic onset of OCD or severely restricted food intake, accompanied by at least two of the following: anxiety, emotional lability or depression, irritability or aggression, behavioural regression, deterioration in school performance, sensory or motor abnormalities, and sleep disturbances (Chang et al., 2015). The criteria for PANDAS additionally require evidence of streptococcal infection.

Many primary care providers are not familiar with PANS and PANDAS. This is not a reflection of poor practice; it reflects a research field that has developed rapidly and whose findings have not yet been fully integrated into general medical training. The family member who brings a written symptom timeline and a printed copy of the diagnostic criteria to a primary care appointment is far more likely to receive a referral than the family member who describes the situation verbally and hopes the provider recognises the pattern.

Action challenge: If sudden-onset symptoms have occurred or are occurring in a child in your family, start a symptom documentation log today. Record the date of onset, the specific symptoms, any preceding illness or infection, and the timeline of any changes since onset. Include any laboratory results that already exist. This log is the most valuable document you will bring to any specialist appointment.

Advocate With Persistence, Not Anger

The PANS and PANDAS diagnostic and treatment pathway is frustrating for most families, and the frustration is legitimate. The medical consensus on these conditions is still developing. Some providers are sceptical of the diagnoses. Waiting times for specialist evaluation can run to months. Insurance coverage for treatment is often contested. The stress level of families in this situation is, as one research team noted, comparable to that of families managing a child with Alzheimer disease (Chang et al., 2015).

The advocacy that works in this context is the same advocacy described in Chapter 7 for school accommodation: specific, documented, and persistent without being confrontational. The family member who arrives at a medical appointment with a written symptom timeline, a list of specific questions, and an explicit request for a specialist referral is more likely to move through the system than the family member who describes their distress and hopes the provider translates that distress into the right next step.

The specific questions worth asking at any primary care appointment include: has the provider considered PANS or PANDAS as a diagnosis, what laboratory tests are appropriate to rule in or rule out a streptococcal or other immune trigger, and what is the referral pathway to a specialist with PANS and PANDAS experience. These questions are not aggressive. They are the questions a medically informed family member asks, and they move the appointment in a more productive direction than a general description of worry.

Lucia's path to the specialist took six months and four different provider conversations. What changed between the third conversation, which ended in another general referral, and the fourth, which produced a referral to the right clinic, was that she had found the diagnostic criteria online and printed them. She did not present them confrontationally. She said: "This is the pattern I have been reading about. Does my son's presentation fit this well enough to warrant an evaluation by someone who specialises in it?" The fourth provider said yes.

Treatment Approaches in Plain Language

Treatment for PANS and PANDAS involves addressing the immune mechanism that is driving the neuropsychiatric symptoms, as well as managing the psychiatric symptoms directly. These are parallel tracks and both require attention.

For the immune mechanism, treatment typically includes antibiotics for documented or suspected bacterial infection, anti-inflammatory medications, and in more severe or refractory cases, immunomodulatory treatments including intravenous immunoglobulin, known as IVIG, or plasmapheresis (Cooperstock et al., 2017). These treatments aim to interrupt the autoimmune process that is producing the neuropsychiatric symptoms. Improvement in symptoms often follows effective treatment of the immune component, though the timeline varies considerably between children.

For the psychiatric symptoms themselves, OCD in PANS and PANDAS is treated with the same exposure and response prevention approach used for classic OCD, and SSRI medications may be used in some cases. The same principles apply here as in Chapter 9: family accommodation of OCD symptoms maintains the OCD, and the treatment approach involves gradual reduction of accommodation alongside direct treatment of the OCD.

The important practical point for families is that effective treatment of PANS and PANDAS typically requires simultaneous attention to both tracks. Treating only the OCD without addressing the immune mechanism may produce limited results. Treating only the immune mechanism without addressing the OCD behavioural patterns may leave the family in an accommodation pattern that maintains the OCD even after the immune driver has resolved.

The Weight of Diagnostic Limbo

The period between recognising that something is dramatically wrong and receiving a clear diagnosis and treatment plan is the period that families consistently describe as the most psychologically costly. It is the period when the child is suffering visibly, when the family member has no framework for understanding what is happening, and when the medical system may not be providing either answers or support. The stress of this period is documented and real.

Lucia described the six months before the PANDAS diagnosis as a period in which she stopped being able to make ordinary decisions. She could not prioritise. She could not concentrate at work. She was not sleeping. She had a child who was frightened and in pain, and she was spending hours each day managing the OCD symptoms because she did not yet know that managing them was making them worse. She was exhausted in a way that did not respond to rest.

Families in this position need two things simultaneously: access to clinical information that moves the diagnostic process forward, and access to personal support that sustains the family member through the process. The second is not a luxury. The family member who is sustained and functional is more effective at advocating, at implementing whatever partial interventions are available, and at being present for the child who needs them most. The family member who has exhausted themselves and isolated themselves in the crisis is less able to do any of these things.

The PANDAS Network at pandasnetwork.org maintains a directory of support groups, specialist providers, and educational resources. Tourette Association of America also provides information on PANS and PANDAS for families already connected to the TS community. These are not substitutes for specialist medical care, but they reduce the isolation of the diagnostic limbo period significantly.

Action challenge: If PANS or PANDAS is a current or suspected diagnosis in your family, identify one specific support resource this week, whether a specialist provider, a support group, or a family contact who has navigated the same process. Write down the contact information. Make one outreach within the next seven days.

Summary

PANS and PANDAS are distinct from classic Tourette Syndrome in one critical way: their onset is sudden and dramatic, typically occurring within 24 to 48 hours of an immune system activation, rather than gradual over months. The primary symptom is severe OCD accompanied by tics, anxiety, and behavioural change, and the condition may account for as many as 25 percent of children diagnosed with OCD and tic disorders. Precise documentation of the onset, the symptom timeline, and the infection history is the most valuable thing a family member can bring to any clinical appointment. Advocacy in the PANS and PANDAS context follows the same specificity principle as school accommodation advocacy: written documentation, specific questions, and explicit referral requests. Treatment addresses both the immune mechanism and the psychiatric symptoms simultaneously. The diagnostic limbo period is genuinely costly, and the family member who maintains their own resources during it is more effective in all the roles the situation requires.

Chapter 11 Partners in the Long Run

Sebastian and Lucia had developed a ritual that began about four years into their relationship, after a period in which the evenings had been reliably difficult and neither of them had understood why.

The difficulty was specific. Sebastian would arrive home from work having suppressed his tics substantially throughout the day, which he did not do deliberately but which happened because the professional environment he worked in was one where his ticcing was visible in ways that made him self-conscious. By the time he was in the car home, the suppression had accumulated into a pressure that required release. He would arrive home, tic intensely for somewhere between thirty and sixty minutes, and then become the version of himself that Lucia had known and chosen and wanted to spend her evenings with.

The problem was that Lucia's evening began at the moment he walked through the door. She had been waiting for him. She had things to say and questions to ask and, on many evenings, something she needed from him that required his full attention. What she was getting instead was forty-five minutes of a person who was, in any practical sense, not yet home even though he was physically present.

Lucia tried several approaches before they found the right one. She tried patience, which she could sustain for about two weeks before the accumulated frustration changed the quality of the patience. She tried using the forty-five minutes for her own tasks, which helped her but did not change the feeling that the evening was starting late every night. She tried, once, saying something about it directly, which produced a conversation that was useful but not a solution.

The solution came from Sebastian. He proposed, tentatively, that the first hour after he got home be designated as a non-conversation zone. Not silence, not isolation, just the absence of anything that required him to be responsive before he was ready to be responsive. He would tic. He would make tea. He would move through the apartment. When the pressure had released, he would find her and they would begin their evening from there.

Lucia said yes. She set an alarm for sixty minutes after his arrival to signal when she could begin. The alarm was not a timer for his performance. It was a reminder of when she had agreed to stop waiting and start doing something else. The distinction was small and everything.

The ritual changed their evenings and consequently their relationship, because the evenings were where the relationship happened. Sebastian felt less guilty and less observed. Lucia felt less impatient and less resentful. Both of them felt more like themselves by the time they were actually together.

The principle of this chapter is that adult partnership with TS requires two things that are in permanent tension: deep understanding of the TS experience, and a clear sense of one's own needs as a separate person within the relationship. The partners who sustain good relationships over the long term are not the ones who subordinate themselves most completely to the TS. They are the ones who find workable forms of each, repeatedly, as the relationship changes.

Intimacy After a Tic-Heavy Day

The suppression cost, described in Chapter 1, has a specific application in adult romantic partnerships that most TS resources do not address. When someone with TS has spent the day managing their tic expression in professional or social settings, they arrive home with a nervous system that has been running on elevated effort for hours. The tics that release at home are the physical evidence of that effort resolving. What is less visible is the cognitive and emotional fatigue that comes with it.

For adult partners, this fatigue has an intimate dimension. The person who is exhausted from a day of suppression and who is releasing that pressure through an evening of intensified ticcing is not, in any meaningful sense, available in the way that intimacy requires. This is not a rejection. It is a physiological fact. Understanding it as a physiological fact rather than as a signal about the relationship is one of the most important reframes available to adult TS partners.

Research on sexual functioning in chronic neurological conditions consistently identifies fatigue as a primary mediating factor in intimate satisfaction (McCabe et al., 2003). For TS specifically, the suppression cost is a form of accumulated fatigue that does not always look like fatigue from the outside. The partner who has been waiting for the evening and who finds that the evening begins in the wrong place regularly may interpret this as a problem with the relationship rather than as a feature of a neurological condition that should have been factored into the evening's design.

Sebastian's ritual addresses this directly, though it was not designed with intimacy in mind. By creating explicit space for the suppression cost to resolve before the relational demands of the evening begin, it produces a partner who is actually present rather than still arriving. The intimate evenings that follow a successful decompression ritual tend to be qualitatively different from the intimate evenings that are attempted before the decompression has happened.

Practical implications: the couple that discusses what the person with TS needs after work before anyone tries to provide it is in a better position than the couple that discovers it through conflict. "What do you need when you get home" is the conversation Sebastian had with Lucia that produced the ritual. It is a conversation worth having at a calm moment before it is needed.

Family Planning Deserves a Real Conversation

The genetics of Tourette Syndrome are well-established and have specific implications for family planning conversations between adult partners. TS is transmitted in an autosomal dominant pattern with variable expressivity and incomplete penetrance. In practical terms, a parent with TS has approximately a 50 percent chance of passing the gene to each biological child, and children who inherit the gene have roughly a 70 to 80 percent chance of expressing some form of tic disorder or related condition (Robertson et al., 2017). Boys are roughly three to four times more likely than girls to express the full TS phenotype.

These statistics are not arguments against having children. They are information that deserves to be part of an informed decision rather than a discovery after the decision has been made. Partners who have not discussed the genetics explicitly are sometimes in the position of learning these numbers after a pregnancy is established and then managing the anxiety of not knowing whether this child will be affected, which is a harder conversation than the one that could have happened earlier.

The most useful version of this conversation happens with the support of a genetic counsellor, who can provide accurate information tailored to the specific couple's situation, address questions about genetic testing, and support the emotional weight of the decision without the pressure of an active pregnancy. Many couples report that the genetic counsellor conversation is significantly less frightening than the one they had been having in their heads without expert input.

Coralie and her partner had the genetic counselling conversation before they married, because TS ran in his family and the question was already present between them even when it was not being spoken. The counsellor normalised it in a way that neither of them had been able to do for themselves, by providing the actual numbers, the actual range of expressions, and the actual life outcomes of adults with TS across the severity range. Coralie said afterwards that she had been imagining the worst version of every statistic in the absence of real information. The real information was different from the imagined version, and manageable in ways the imagined version was not.

Action challenge: If family planning is relevant to your partnership, have the genetics conversation before it is required by circumstances rather than after. If you have not yet spoken with a genetic counsellor, find one with experience in neurogenetic conditions and make one appointment. You do not need to have any specific decision to make. You need the information in order to make it well.

Supporting Without Caretaking

The line between supporting a partner and caretaking a partner is one of the most practically difficult things to locate in a long-term TS relationship. It is also one of the most important. Partners who cross from support into caretaking tend to build a relational dynamic in which the person with TS becomes increasingly dependent and the partner becomes increasingly resentful, neither of which outcome is good for either person.

The distinction, in practical terms, is about agency. Support provides information, resources, and presence while leaving the person with TS as the decision-maker and the actor. Caretaking removes decisions and actions from the person with TS and performs them on their behalf, initially out of love and efficiency, eventually out of habit.

Julian and Mateo's grocery shopping story, which appeared in Chapter 4, is the clearest example in this book of caretaking that had begun as support. Julian took over a task that Mateo found difficult. Over time, the task became Julian's. The difficulty was never worked through because it did not need to be; Julian had made it disappear. Mateo became someone who did not grocery shop, not because he could not but because he had never been asked to try again after the first difficult attempt.

The corrective is not to withdraw support suddenly. It is to periodically review, together, which supports are still being provided because the person with TS needs them and which are being provided because the system has settled into them. This review is a conversation that requires honesty from both people: the partner about what they are providing, and the person with TS about what they actually need versus what they have become accustomed to receiving.

Hugo and Noemi had a version of this review after Noemi realised she had been sending work emails on Hugo's behalf for months. He had asked her to help with one specific email at a point when his ADHD-related executive function difficulties were making the task nearly impossible. She had helped, the email had been sent, and at some point the responsibility for certain categories of correspondence had shifted to her without either of them formally deciding it. The conversation when she named this was uncomfortable. The adjustment that followed was gradual. Hugo began managing his own correspondence again, with a specific structure Noemi helped him design, rather than having Noemi manage it for him.

The Difference Between Partner and Therapist

Partners of people with TS sometimes find themselves performing a quasi-therapeutic function in the relationship: providing psychoeducation, offering cognitive reframes during difficult moments, managing the emotional processing of TS-related experiences, and generally doing the emotional work of treatment in the absence of professional support. This role is exhausting, is beyond the scope of any partnership, and tends to damage the intimate quality of the relationship over time.

The difference between the partner role and the therapist rolc is not merely professional. It is relational. A therapist who provides psychological support does so within a bounded, paid, non-mutual relationship. A partner who provides the same support is doing so within a relationship that requires mutuality, which means their own needs are also in the room. When those needs are consistently subordinated to the therapeutic function, the relationship eventually stops being a partnership and starts being a care arrangement.

The way out is referral to actual professional support. This means actively identifying and supporting access to a therapist, CBIT practitioner, or psychiatrist rather than filling the gap their absence creates. It means being honest when the conversation that is happening is beyond what a partner can appropriately provide. And it means maintaining the relational qualities, curiosity, playfulness, partnership, and the particular kind of presence that is distinctly not therapeutic, that make the partnership worth having.

Couples therapy, when both people are willing to engage with it, can be a useful space for working through the dynamics that develop in long-term TS partnerships. The most useful therapists for this work are those with experience in chronic illness or neurodevelopmental conditions, who can provide psychoeducation to both partners while holding the relational dynamics rather than treating the TS as the only subject.

Action challenge: Write down the five things you most need from your partnership, in your own words, without reference to TS. Then, for each one, note whether that need is currently being met. If two or more are not being met because the TS management demands are taking up the space where those things would otherwise happen, name this in a conversation with your partner at a calm moment. The naming is the beginning of finding the balance.

Summary

Adult partnership with TS requires understanding the suppression cost as a physiological reality that shapes the evenings, the intimate life, and the emotional availability of the person with TS on any given day. Family planning conversations about TS genetics are better had with a genetic counsellor before they are required by circumstances. The line between supporting a partner and caretaking them is crossed when agency is systematically removed from the person with TS, and periodic review of which supports are still necessary prevents this from happening invisibly. The partner role and the therapist role are distinct, and the partnership is healthier when professional support does the therapeutic work and the partnership does the relational work.

Chapter 12 Everyone in the Family

The year Martin turned eleven, his younger sister Margot told a boy at school that her brother had Tourette Syndrome and the boy had laughed, and Margot had said, in a clear and steady voice, that it was a neurological condition that affected his brain and was not his fault and was not something he could control, and would the boy please stop. The boy had stopped. Margot was eight years old.

Clara heard about this from her daughter's teacher, who had been standing close enough to overhear. The teacher said she had been impressed by both the composure and the accuracy of the explanation. Clara, when she was alone later, cried.

She cried because it had not occurred to her that Margot was carrying information that precise. She had spoken to Margot about Martin's TS, of course, multiple times, using words she had calibrated for an eight-year-old. She had not known whether the words had landed in a useful way or whether they had become one more piece of background noise in a household where the background noise was already significant. She had been so focused on what Martin needed that she had not clearly seen what Margot was doing with what she had been given.

Margot had been making herself into someone who could defend her brother. She had filed away what she had been told and had prepared, in whatever private way eight-year-olds prepare, for the moment when it would be needed. She had done this quietly, alongside the jealousy and the occasional resentment that Clara also knew were there, because children contain more than one thing at once and siblings of children with significant conditions are no exception.

The sibling experience in a TS household is one of the most overlooked and most consequential aspects of family life with TS. Siblings absorb the household's attention patterns, the emotional weather of tic episodes and rage attacks, the family's social adjustments and avoidances, and the conversations their parents have at the kitchen table when they think the children are not listening. They develop opinions, loyalties, competencies, and resentments in response to all of this, and most of them do not have anyone asking them what the experience is like from where they stand.

The principle of this chapter is that the wider family system, including siblings, grandparents, and extended family members, does not sort itself out passively. It responds to what is given to it. The family that gives siblings accurate information, appropriate expectations, and genuine attention to their own experience produces siblings who are allies. The family that gives siblings none of these things produces a different outcome.

Siblings Need Their Own Information

The age-appropriate explanation of TS for siblings is one of the most practically useful tools a parent can develop, and most parents either do not develop it or develop it imprecisely. The precision matters because the explanation that is given shapes how the sibling understands, and therefore how they respond to, what they observe in the household.

For children under six, the explanation that works best is physical, concrete, and brief. "Martin's brain sends messages to his body that make him move and make sounds he can't stop. It doesn't hurt him. He can't help it." This is sufficient. Young children are not seeking a neurological account. They are seeking enough information to understand that what they see is not alarming and is not their fault.

For children between seven and twelve, more nuance is appropriate. "Martin has a condition called Tourette Syndrome. His brain is wired in a way that makes him tic, which is a word for the movements and sounds you see. He also has some other things that come along with it, like it being hard for him to control his attention sometimes, and he can have big feelings that come out fast. None of this is because he is bad at controlling himself. His brain works differently." This explanation gives the sibling a framework for understanding not just the tics but the full TS-Plus picture at an accessible level.

For adolescents, honesty about complexity serves better than simplification. Adolescent siblings are often managing their own social identity alongside the family identity, and they frequently have specific concerns that are not about the TS itself but about how the TS appears to their peers and affects their own social standing. An honest conversation that acknowledges this rather than dismissing it, and that discusses practical strategies for managing it, is more useful than a clinical explanation alone.

Eloise's daughter, who is now fifteen, has had three different versions of the explanation of her brother's TS over the years. The first version, at age five, was the physical and brief one. The second, at age nine, added the TS-Plus context. The third, at thirteen, was a conversation in which Eloise asked her daughter what questions she had that had not been answered, and the answer surprised her. Her daughter's most pressing question was not about the neuroscience. It was about whether her brother's TS would mean that Eloise would always be more worried about him than about her. They talked for two hours.

The Attention Imbalance Is Real and Must Be Named

The sibling of a child with TS-Plus is living in a household where significant parental attention, energy, and resources are directed toward the sibling with the most complex needs. This is not a failure of parenting. It is an arithmetical reality of having a child with a condition that makes ongoing and often unpredictable demands. But it is an experience that must be acknowledged directly rather than hoped around.

Research on siblings of children with chronic conditions consistently finds that the siblings are at elevated risk for anxiety, depression, and adjustment difficulties when they perceive the attention imbalance as permanent and unnamed (Sharpe & Rossiter, 2002). The same research finds that siblings who feel that their own experience is acknowledged and that they have access to the parent when they need it, regardless of the asymmetry in overall allocation, show better outcomes. The variable is not the imbalance itself. It is whether the imbalance is invisible or named.

Naming the imbalance is a specific act, not a general acknowledgement. It sounds like: "I know that a lot of our family's energy goes toward managing Gabriel's TS. I know that is not always easy for you. I want to hear what the hard parts are." It does not sound like: "You know we love you both equally." The second statement may be true but it does not address what the sibling is experiencing. The first statement invites the actual conversation.

Paloma had been making the second statement for two years before she made the first one. Her elder daughter's response to the first statement, on a Thursday evening in the kitchen, was to start talking and not stop for forty minutes. Paloma had not known her daughter had that much to say. She had not asked in a way that made it possible to say.

Grandparents Require Patient Repetition

The grandparent who believes that Tourette Syndrome is a behavioural problem caused by insufficient discipline is not an unusual figure in TS families. They appear across cultures, across socioeconomic contexts, and across family structures. They are often people who love the child deeply and whose love expresses itself through the offer of solutions that have not worked and would not work. Their explanatory framework for the condition is wrong, and it is entrenched in ways that rational argument rarely shifts.

What shifts grandparents, in the experience of many TS families, is repetition and demonstration rather than argument. The itch-and-scratch metaphor from Chapter 5 is the right level of explanation for most grandparents: physical, immediate, non-clinical, and requiring no prior knowledge of neurology to understand. The grandparent who has heard this explanation once may not fully integrate it. The grandparent who has heard it three times, and who has watched the grandchild do something impressive or funny in between, and who has seen the parent respond calmly to a tic episode rather than with alarm, begins to update their model.

Oscar's grandmother had been the most sceptical family member at the time of his childhood diagnosis and had become, by his early adulthood, one of his most vocal advocates in her social circle. The shift had happened over about eight years and had not involved a single conversation that Oscar or his parents identified as the turning point. It had happened through accumulated contact, repeated low-key explanations, and being present during moments when Oscar handled his TS with such evident competence that the character-flaw model simply ceased to hold together.

Time is the most reliable tool with grandparents who resist. Patience is the posture. And the occasional, gently delivered correction of a specific wrong statement is more effective than a general challenge to the grandparent's entire framework.

Family Meetings Work When They Have Structure

The family meeting about TS, when it happens in an unstructured way, tends to produce one of two outcomes: either the person with TS dominates as the subject and everyone else manages their feelings about that, or the person with TS disengages because they feel they are being assessed rather than included. Neither outcome serves the family.

The family meeting that produces useful outcomes is the one with a specific and limited agenda, explicit roles, and a clear signal for when it is over. The agenda might be as simple as: we are going to spend thirty minutes talking about how things are going in our family, and each person will have five minutes to say something without being interrupted. The roles are: who facilitates, who keeps time, who ensures that the youngest person in the room has had a turn. The signal for when it is over is the end of the thirty minutes, not the resolution of every topic.

Hugo's family had tried and abandoned the unstructured family meeting several times before they tried the structured version. The difference, he said, was that the structured version did not feel like a meeting about him. It felt like a meeting that included him, which was an entirely different experience.

Action challenge: Write three brief explanations of TS for the people in your extended family system who need one: one for a young child, one for an older child or adolescent, and one for an adult who has not yet understood the condition accurately. Keep each one under five sentences. Use no clinical language. Read each one aloud. Adjust until they feel natural. These are your working explanations for the next year.

Summary

Siblings in a TS household are absorbing the family's full experience of the condition, including the attention patterns, the emotional weather, and the practical adjustments, and they need accurate, age-appropriate information and genuine attention to their own experience in order to do this well. The attention imbalance that is a mathematical reality in TS families produces better sibling outcomes when it is named directly rather than hoped around. Grandparents and extended family members who resist the TS explanation are best approached through patient repetition, physical metaphors, and demonstrated competence over time rather than through argument. Family meetings produce useful outcomes when they have a specific structure, explicit roles, and a clear time limit, and when the person with TS is included rather than merely discussed.

Chapter 13 What the Screen Gets Wrong

Paloma's son Gabriel had been doing well. His tics were manageable, his CBIT work was progressing, and his school, for the first time since his diagnosis, had a written accommodation plan that was being followed consistently. Paloma had spent two years building those conditions, one difficult conversation at a time. She had been, cautiously, beginning to feel something like steadiness.

Then she got a phone call from the school's special educational needs coordinator.

The coordinator's tone was measured but Paloma could hear something careful underneath it. She explained that one of Gabriel's classroom teachers had watched, over the preceding weekend, a documentary-style video about Tourette Syndrome that had been widely shared on social media. The video, which had several million views, focused almost entirely on individuals with coprolalia. It included dramatic footage of outbursts in public settings, commentary from a clinical expert who was given approximately forty seconds of screen time, and a host narrator who repeatedly used the word "bizarre" and the phrase "sufferers who cannot control themselves."

The teacher had come to school on Monday with a revised understanding of what Tourette Syndrome was. The revised understanding bore little resemblance to Gabriel's actual experience. The teacher had approached Gabriel at the start of the morning session and, with evident concern, asked whether he ever had the urge to say bad words.

Gabriel was eleven. He did not have coprolalia. He had never had coprolalia. He had spent two years, with his mother's support, learning to explain his tics matter-of-factly to the adults around him, and this teacher had undone a significant portion of that work in a single misguided question.

Paloma drove to the school that afternoon and had a conversation with the coordinator that was, by her account, one of the more controlled performances of her adult life. She brought printed materials. She named the specific ways the video had misrepresented TS. She made a request, in writing, that the accommodation plan be reviewed with all teaching staff and that no further direct questioning of Gabriel about his symptoms happen without her prior involvement.

The coordinator agreed to all of it. She said, genuinely, that she had not known the video was circulating. She asked what a reliable source would look like.

Paloma thought about that question for a long time on the drive home. She had spent two years learning how to answer it. What she had not expected was that she would need to teach the answer to the people who were supposed to be helping her son.

The media landscape around Tourette Syndrome has never been more crowded or more confusing. There is more public attention on TS than at any point in the condition's history, and more misinformation circulating than there has ever been access to reliable information. The principle of this chapter is that media literacy about TS is not optional for the families of people with TS. It is a survival skill. The family member who cannot evaluate a source, correct a specific misrepresentation, or explain why the coprolalia stereotype misrepresents most people with TS is inadequately equipped for the information environment their family now operates in.

The Coprolalia Stereotype Is Not a Portrait of TS

Coprolalia, the involuntary vocalisation of obscene or taboo words, affects approximately 10 to 20 percent of people with Tourette Syndrome (Robertson et al., 2017). This means that between 80 and 90 percent of people with TS do not have it. The entertainment and media industries have repeatedly represented coprolalia as the defining feature of Tourette Syndrome, producing a population of viewers who believe that TS is synonymous with involuntary swearing and who apply this belief to every person with TS they encounter, including those who have never produced an obscene vocalisation in their lives.

The costs of this misrepresentation are specific and documented. People with TS who do not have coprolalia regularly encounter doubt about their diagnosis from people who expected something more dramatic. People with TS who do have coprolalia encounter a different problem: they embody the stereotype that others seek to correct, which makes them doubly marginalised within a community already working against public misunderstanding (Zito, 2025). And the families of both groups encounter a third problem: they must manage the gap between the public's media-formed understanding and the reality of their loved one's actual experience, in every new social and institutional setting.

The correction is short and must become automatic. "Most people with Tourette Syndrome don't have coprolalia. The media focuses on it because it's dramatic, but it affects fewer than one in five people with the condition." This sentence, said without defensiveness and with the confidence of someone who has checked the research, closes most misunderstandings in a single exchange.

Eloise used a version of this sentence so frequently in Gabriel's early school years that she once counted the number of times she said it in a single week. She stopped at seven. After that she stopped counting and simply said it, automatically, whenever the word Tourette produced the particular expression in a stranger's face that meant they were already imagining something that had nothing to do with her son.

The TikTok Tic Surge Requires Careful Handling

In 2020 and the years that followed, clinicians across multiple countries documented a significant increase in presentations of what came to be called functional tic-like behaviours, primarily in adolescent girls with no prior tic history (Pringsheim et al., 2021). These presentations shared surface features with Tourette Syndrome, including motor movements and vocalisations, but differed in several clinically meaningful ways: sudden onset in adolescence rather than childhood, female predominance rather than the roughly four-to-one male ratio typical of TS, absence of the premonitory urge in many cases, and a close temporal relationship with exposure to tic-related content on social media platforms, particularly TikTok.

The research on this phenomenon is ongoing and its interpretation is contested. What is established is that functional tic-like behaviours are a genuine clinical phenomenon, are not simply copycat behaviour in any dismissive sense, and are best understood as a form of functional neurological disorder that is distinct from Tourette Syndrome and responds to different treatment approaches (Pringsheim et al., 2021). What is also established is that the widespread coverage of this phenomenon has created a secondary problem for families of people with genuine TS diagnoses.

The secondary problem is this: the post-2020 surge in tic presentations has made the question of whether a given person's tics are "real" or "TikTok tics" a more common one in clinical and educational settings than it should be. Teachers, employers, and even some medical providers who have read articles about the functional tic surge may approach a person with a longstanding TS diagnosis with a scepticism that the diagnosis does not warrant. Paloma's teacher, who had watched a video about coprolalia rather than about functional tics, represents one version of this problem.

The teacher who has read about TikTok tics and applies that framework to a child who has had motor tics since age seven represents another.

The family member's practical tool here is the developmental history. Tourette Syndrome begins in childhood, typically before age 12, with motor tics preceding vocal tics, and the history is usually clear and documentable (Robertson et al., 2017). A person with a genuine TS diagnosis has a timeline, a clinical record, and in most cases a pattern of waxing and waning that has been observed over years. This history distinguishes the TS diagnosis from a functional tic presentation that began in adolescence, and it is the most effective piece of information to present when the distinction is being questioned.

Action challenge: Write a brief documented history of the TS diagnosis in your family: the age of first tic onset, the progression of tic types over time, the formal diagnosis date and provider, and any significant treatment history. Keep this document somewhere accessible. It is the most direct response to any scepticism about the diagnosis's validity.

Evaluate Sources Before Acting On Them

The volume of TS-related content available online is high, the quality is inconsistent, and the stakes of acting on wrong information are real. A family member who modifies their home behaviour, their communication approach, or their treatment decisions based on a YouTube video or a social media post that does not reflect the research literature is not being helped by the internet's abundance of TS content. They are being misled by it.

Five questions that produce reliable source evaluation, applied in sequence:

First, who produces this content? Academic medical centres, established advocacy organisations such as the Tourette Association of America, NJCTS, Tourettes Action UK, and the

CDC TS resource pages produce information that is reviewed and updated against the research literature. Individual social media creators, however genuine their experience, produce information that reflects their own history rather than the clinical range.

Second, are citations provided for factual claims? Any source that makes a statistical or clinical claim without indicating where the claim comes from cannot be verified. This does not mean the claim is wrong. It means the reader cannot check it.

Third, when was this content produced? TS treatment guidelines have changed meaningfully in the past decade, particularly with the introduction of CBIT as the recommended first-line treatment in 2019. Content older than five to seven years may reflect an outdated treatment framework.

Fourth, does the content reflect the full TS picture or primarily one feature? Any resource that discusses TS exclusively through the lens of coprolalia, or exclusively through the lens of the TikTok tic surge, is giving a partial account of a condition that is considerably more varied than any single feature suggests.

Fifth, does the content encourage family members to seek professional support or to substitute for it? Reliable resources consistently emphasise that TS management requires professional evaluation and treatment. Resources that discourage professional engagement or position themselves as replacements for it warrant particular caution.

Noemi developed a version of this evaluation process after a period during which she had made several household changes based on content from a TS influencer account that was, on closer inspection, drawing almost all of its clinical claims from a single self-published book that pre-dated the CBIT evidence base. The changes she had made were not harmful, but they were not the most useful changes she could have made, and she had not known that until she looked more carefully at the source.

Action challenge: Take one piece of TS-related content you have acted on or shared in the past six months, whether an article, a video, or an online post, and run it through the five questions above. Write down what the evaluation produces. If the source falls short of two or more of the five questions, identify the closest reliable source for the same information and note where to find it next time.

Reliable Sources Are a Short List

The family member who has five reliable sources bookmarked and checked regularly is better resourced than the family member who has fifty sources of varying quality. The short list of reliable TS information sources is not exhaustive, but it is consistently trustworthy.

The Tourette Association of America, at tourette.org, maintains clinical information, school and workplace resources, a CBIT provider directory, and family guides that are updated against the research literature. The New Jersey Center for Tourette Syndrome and Associated Disorders, at njcts.org, provides educator and parent resources that are particularly strong on school advocacy and the TS-Plus profile. Tourettes Action UK, at tourettes.org.uk, provides resources calibrated to the UK educational and healthcare context. The CDC's Tourette Syndrome pages, at cdc.gov/tourette, provide epidemiological data and evidence summaries that are free from commercial interest. The PANDAS Network, at pandasnetwork.org, provides the most reliable family-accessible information on PANS and PANDAS.

Each of these organisations publishes information that can be shared with teachers, employers, family members, and medical providers who need to be educated about TS. They are not entertainment. They are reliable reference material, and treating them as such, returning to them when new information is needed rather than turning to the most recent social media content, is the most reliable way a family member can stay accurately informed.

Help Your Loved One Navigate Online TS Content

The person with TS in your family is also encountering TS content online, and their experience of that content is different from yours in specific ways. When a teenager with TS watches a video that misrepresents the condition as comedic material, or encounters comments on a creator's TS-related post that reduce the condition to a punchline, the impact is not merely informational. It is personal. The misrepresentation is of them.

The family member who can discuss what the person with TS is encountering online, without alarm and with the factual tools to correct what is incorrect, is providing something valuable: a counterweight to an information environment that frequently distorts rather than informs. This is not a single conversation. It is an ongoing one, as the content the person with TS encounters changes and as their capacity to interpret and respond to it develops.

Felix, now in his early thirties, has said that the most useful thing his parents did when he was in his late teens was not protect him from the media's representation of TS but talk to him about it directly. When a film character's TS was played for laughs, his father would ask what he thought of it. When a news article described TS in language that did not match Felix's experience, his mother would note the discrepancy without dramatising it. They did not resolve the misrepresentation. They gave him a framework for encountering it without internalising it as fact.

Summary

The coprolalia stereotype affects 10 to 20 percent of people with TS but represents nearly all media portrayals of the condition; the correction is short, factual, and must become automatic. The TikTok tic surge produced a documented clinical phenomenon distinct from genuine TS, and the developmental history of a TS diagnosis is the most effective tool when the validity of the diagnosis is questioned. Source evaluation using five consistent questions, who produces it, whether citations are provided, when it was produced, what portion of the TS picture it reflects, and whether it encourages professional support, reduces the risk of acting on unreliable information. The short list of reliable TS organisations is worth knowing and returning to. And the person with TS benefits from a family member who can discuss the media's misrepresentation of the condition factually rather than avoiding the subject.

Chapter 14 The Road Gets Easier

Oscar had not been sure, at fifteen, that he would make it to twenty.

This was not a dramatic statement. He did not mean it dramatically. He meant it in the specific, practical sense that he could not, at fifteen, construct a mental image of himself as a functioning adult. The tics were at their most intense during those years, his most visible and most socially costly, and he had developed the habit of projecting his current experience forward indefinitely, so that what he saw when he tried to imagine his future was simply more of what was happening now, forever.

His mother knew this without being told. She could read it in the specific way he had stopped talking about future plans, in the careful flatness he maintained when school discussions turned to university or career. She did not challenge the flatness directly. She had learned, over fifteen years of living with Oscar, that challenging it directly produced withdrawal rather than engagement. Instead, she started telling him stories about adults she had met through the Tourette Association who had lives that worked. She did this occasionally and without pressure, over the course of about a year, so that the information arrived without the weight of being delivered.

One of those adults was a man who had been a research scientist. Another had been a teacher. A third ran a small business that had been operating for twelve years. None of them had been cured. All of them had tics that were less severe in their thirties than they had been in their teens, which was something Oscar's neurologist had also told him but which had landed differently when he heard it from someone who had been where he was.

The natural history of Tourette Syndrome is one of the most genuinely hopeful facts about the condition, and one of the facts most consistently missing from the information families receive at the point of diagnosis. Tic severity in TS follows a well-documented developmental trajectory: onset in early childhood, gradual increase through middle childhood, peak severity typically between the ages of 10 and 12, followed for most people by a period of gradual reduction through adolescence and into early adulthood (Leckman et al., 1998). By adulthood, approximately one-third of people with TS have tics that are minimal or no longer clinically significant, one-third have mild residual tics that do not substantially impair functioning, and one-third continue to have tics that are moderate to severe (Bloch & Leckman, 2009).

This is not a guarantee. It is a population-level pattern with individual variation. But for families who are in the most difficult years of the tic peak, knowing that the pattern exists and that it applies to the majority of people with TS changes the emotional experience of the present. The present is not the permanent. Most children with TS at their worst between the ages of 10 and 13 are not at their worst in their twenties.

The principle of this chapter is that understanding the natural history of TS gives families both a realistic long-term picture and a different quality of attention to the present, because the present is finite in a way that the crisis years can make it impossible to feel.

The Tic Peak Is Usually Not the Permanent State

The research on tic severity over time is consistent enough to be presented as a reliable expectation rather than a tentative hope. Studies following individuals with TS from childhood through adulthood have found that tic severity scores peak in early adolescence and decline meaningfully in late adolescence and early adulthood for the majority of participants (Leckman et al., 1998; Bloch & Leckman, 2009). The decline is not universal, and the TS-Plus conditions, particularly OCD and ADHD, often persist with less reduction than the tics themselves. But the tic trajectory, for most people, improves.

What this means practically for families at the tic peak is that treatment decisions, accommodation strategies, and household adjustments made in the worst years do not need to be permanent. The CBIT work done during adolescence builds skills that remain available even when the tic severity they were designed for has reduced. The school accommodations that protect academic performance at twelve do not necessarily reflect what will be needed at eighteen. The family member who understands the trajectory can plan in phases rather than indefinitely, which is a less exhausting way to manage a condition that sometimes makes indefinite planning feel impossible.

Clara had been managing the most intensive phase of Martin's TS for four years when his neurologist mentioned, almost in passing at a routine appointment, that Martin's tic peak was likely somewhere behind them. She sat with that sentence for a while. She had not known they had been at a peak. She had been living inside it, which made its edges impossible to see. The neurologist showed her the data on tic severity trajectories, which she had encountered before in articles but which looked different when placed next to her son's current profile. The peak was behind them. The shape of the future had just changed.

Action challenge: If you have not had an explicit conversation with the treating clinician about the natural history of TS and what to expect over the next five to ten years, schedule that conversation before the next routine appointment. Write down three specific questions: where is this person likely to be at twenty, which of the current TS-Plus challenges are most likely to persist even as tics improve, and what does the transition to adult care look like in this healthcare context?

Prepare for Adulthood While It Is Still Ahead

The transition from child to adult services in any chronic neurological condition is a period of elevated risk for disruption, and TS is no exception. The specialist paediatrician who has managed the condition since childhood does not have an adult counterpart who automatically receives the handoff. The school accommodations that have been carefully built over years do not transfer automatically to higher education or employment. The family member who has been the primary coordinator of services and advocate for access does not have a formalised successor.

Planning for this transition is most effective when it begins earlier than it feels necessary. For most families, the transition conversation should start no later than age 15 or 16, which gives two to three years for the young person with TS to begin practising the self-advocacy skills they will need to manage their own condition in adult settings.

Self-advocacy in TS has a specific curriculum. The young person needs to be able to name their diagnosis and its primary manifestations in plain language, to request accommodations in their own words rather than through a parent's mediation, to identify when a situation is not working and communicate that to a relevant adult, and to access their own clinical records and understand their treatment history. None of these things develop automatically. They develop through practice, in progressively more independent settings, with the family member stepping gradually back from the coordination role they have held.

Hugo began this process with his parents when he was seventeen, after a conversation in which his father said something that stayed with him: "We've been managing this for you for a long time. We'd like to start helping you manage it for yourself." It was not a withdrawal of support. It was a reframing of what support was now supposed to look like. Hugo said it was the most useful thing his father said to him during adolescence, and he said it from the position of someone who had not, at seventeen, fully appreciated it.

When TS Remains Significantly Impairing in Adulthood

For the minority of adults whose TS remains moderate to severe, the long-term planning described above is more urgent and more complex. This population needs adult specialist care, which means a movement disorder neurologist or psychiatrist with TS expertise rather than a general adult neurology practice. It may mean continued and potentially adjusted CBIT work. It may mean ongoing workplace accommodations that become a permanent feature of professional life rather than a temporary support.

The family members of adults with persistent severe TS face a specific adjustment: the mental model built around the tic peak and the natural improvement trajectory does not describe their loved one. They need a different frame, one that acknowledges the condition as a permanent feature of adult life without treating it as a catastrophe, and one that identifies the specific supports that make adult life with significant TS workable rather than the supports that might have been appropriate during childhood.

Valeria, who had managed Felix's medication history on a spreadsheet for three years, had expected by his mid-thirties that the tics would have reduced substantially. They had reduced, but not as much as the population-level data had suggested they might. Felix was, by most measures, functioning well: he had work, a relationship, a social life, and a CBIT-supported tic management approach that was considerably more effective than anything available to him in his twenties. He was not the severity-peak version of himself. He was also not tic-free. Valeria had needed time to adjust to the distance between the outcome she had hoped for and the outcome they were actually in. The outcome they were actually in was manageable. It took her a while to see it that way.

Grieve What Was Hard and Move Forward

The difficult years of a TS family's experience, and most families have some years that qualify as genuinely difficult, leave a residue that is worth addressing rather than simply moving past. Parents who spent years in hypervigilance around their child's tics, in conflict with schools, in anxiety about public episodes and the long-term future, do not emerge from those years without some cost. The cost is real and should be acknowledged.

The acknowledgement is not a dwelling. It is a recognition that significant sustained difficulty has a psychological weight that does not lift automatically when the circumstances improve. The family that moves from the crisis years into a more stable phase without pausing to name what the crisis years were like may find the weight surfacing later, in ways that are harder to attribute to their actual source.

Zoe, whose relationship with Gabriel's OCD had required her to change deeply held instincts about how to help her child, described the period after the change as one of the stranger experiences of her adult life. The mornings were easier. The OCD was genuinely less severe. She was, by observable measures, in a better situation. She was also tired in a way that the better situation had not immediately resolved. She told a friend that she felt like someone who had been bracing for a long time and had not yet learned how to stop bracing.

This is a common enough experience in TS families that it deserves to be named: the transition from crisis to stability does not feel like the relief it looked like from the outside. The body and the mind that adapted to the crisis do not de-adapt immediately. Some deliberate attention to that de-adaptation, through one's own therapy, through conversation with others who

of them to the sustained effort of loving someone with TS in the specific way that TS requires.

The principle of this chapter is simple and often resisted: the family member's own condition is a clinical variable in the TS household. Not a moral consideration, not a luxury, not something to be attended to once the more pressing needs have been addressed. A variable, in the same sense that suppression cost and OCD accommodation are variables, that affects the household's overall function. The family member who is depleted provides qualitatively different support from the family member who has adequate resources. The difference is measurable and it matters.

Caregiver Burnout Has Specific Signs

Burnout in TS family members does not typically announce itself. It develops gradually, across months or years, through the accumulation of a sustained effort that is rarely named as effort because it is simply what love requires in this context. The person experiencing it often does not recognise it as burnout because they are, in most cases, still functioning: still going to work, still managing the household, still showing up for appointments and school meetings and the daily negotiations that TS-Plus demands.

The signs that tend to appear before the person recognises what is happening: physical symptoms without clear medical cause, including persistent tension, headaches, and disrupted sleep that is not explained by the person with TS's own sleep issues. A reduction in the ability to feel engaged with activities that previously produced enjoyment. A shortening of the patience available for interactions that have nothing to do with TS, because the patience reservoir is being used elsewhere. And the specific emotional pattern that researchers have called compassion fatigue: a dulling of the emotional responsiveness that usually motivates the caregiving, so that the person provides care through habit and obligation rather than through the connection that began the relationship.

Research on caregivers of individuals with chronic neurological conditions consistently finds elevated rates of anxiety, depression, and reduced quality of life in the caregivers themselves, and consistently finds that caregivers are less likely than the people they care for to seek or receive support for these outcomes (Majeske et al., 2018). The combination of these two findings produces a population that is significantly affected and significantly under-resourced, quietly, in households that are otherwise highly focused on clinical management.

Noemi recognised her own pattern when she completed a standard caregiver wellbeing questionnaire as part of a research study she had enrolled in through a TS family network. The questionnaire asked about her emotional state, her relationships, her activities, and her sense of being supported. She answered honestly because there was no one in the room who knew her. Her scores on several subscales were significantly below the normative range. She had not known there was a normative range for this kind of thing. She had thought her experience was simply what it was to be the person she was in the situation she was in.

Action challenge: Rate yourself, right now, on four dimensions, from one (significantly depleted) to ten (fully resourced): energy available for your own needs, resentment in the caregiving relationship, joy experienced in an average week outside of TS-related contexts, and felt connection to people and activities that are entirely your own. Write the scores down. If two or more are below five, the situation is worth attending to with more deliberateness than it has received.

Secondary Stigma Has a Real Cost

The concept of secondary stigma, introduced briefly in Chapter 6, deserves more direct attention in the context of the caregiver's own experience. Secondary stigma is the social cost experienced by family members of people with stigmatised conditions, through their association with the condition rather than through any symptoms of their own.

For partners and parents of people with TS, secondary stigma operates in several ways. The parent who is asked, repeatedly, what they did that caused their child's tics. The partner who receives looks in public during a tic episode that include a component of assessment: what is wrong with them that they are with this person? The family member who stops bringing the person with TS to certain social events because the management of other people's reactions has become too costly. The friend who drifts away because the relationship has become too hard to sustain in its previous form.

These experiences accumulate. They produce a specific kind of social fatigue, a wariness about new environments and new relationships, that is distinct from ordinary social anxiety because it is based on a realistic assessment of what tends to happen. The family member who has been the subject of secondary stigma repeatedly is not being paranoid. They are being accurate, and their accuracy comes from experience.

The most effective response to secondary stigma, at the individual level, is the same media literacy and corrective communication described in Chapter 13: the short, factual, non-defensive response that provides accurate information without invitation for extended debate. At the family level, it is the cultivation of a social network that includes at minimum a few people who understand TS well enough that the family member does not need to manage others' responses in their presence. The TS family community, both in local support groups and in online networks attached to the Tourette Association and similar organisations, provides this kind of contact in a form that is available to most families regardless of geography.

Build Support Before It Is Urgently Needed

The family member who waits until they are in crisis before building a support network is building it under the most difficult conditions. The family member who builds it before the crisis has somewhere to go when the crisis arrives.

Support for TS family members takes several forms, and the most effective combination typically includes more than one. Peer support, through contact with other family members navigating the same experience, provides the specific understanding that friends and family outside the TS context often cannot. Individual therapy, with a therapist who understands chronic illness and neurodevelopmental conditions, provides the professional support that is distinct from peer support in its scope and depth. And the maintenance of at least some activities, relationships, and contexts that have nothing to do with TS provides the ongoing reminder that the caregiving relationship is one dimension of a full life rather than the whole of it.

Finding a therapist with TS-specific knowledge is not always easy. It is worth asking the CBIT therapist or the treating neurologist for referrals. TS advocacy organisations sometimes maintain referral lists for family members as well as for the people with TS. If no specialist is available, a therapist experienced in chronic illness caregiving is a reasonable second option. The knowledge they lack about TS specifically can be provided by the family member. The understanding of sustained caregiving that they bring to the work cannot be substituted.

Coralie had been in therapy for six months before she mentioned TS in a session. She had been seeing the therapist for her own anxiety, which had been present in her life before her partner's diagnosis and which had intensified significantly after it. The therapist had not asked about chronic illness or caregiving in the initial intake. Coralie had not thought to volunteer it because she had not yet understood that the anxiety she was experiencing and the TS caregiving she was doing were related in the specific way that they were. The session in which she made the connection was, by her account, the most useful session she had in the eighteen months she worked with that therapist.

Attending to Yourself Models Something Important

There is one aspect of the family member's own wellbeing that is not merely about the family member and that is worth naming: the way the family member manages their own difficult emotional experiences is the most visible model available to the person with TS for how difficult emotional experiences can be managed.

A person with TS who grows up watching a parent respond to difficulty with stoic concealment learns that stoic concealment is the appropriate response to difficulty. A person with TS who grows up watching a parent seek support when support is needed, rest when rest is needed, and maintain relationships and activities of their own alongside the demands of caregiving, learns that these things are compatible with love and responsibility.

This is not an argument for performing wellness. It is an argument for actually attending to your own experience, partly because you are worth attending to, and partly because the person with TS who will eventually need to manage their own experience of a demanding condition is watching how you do it.

Marcel said this about Ines, in a conversation they had when he was considerably better than he had been, when the CBIT was working and the medication was stable and the spreadsheet was no longer necessary: he said that the thing she had done that helped him most was not the three sentences in the car or the treatment summary at the neurologist's appointment. It was that she had, at some point, stopped being afraid. He could not remember when it happened. He only knew that it had, and that the change in her had changed something in how he moved through each day.

Action challenge: Identify one specific thing you have been consistently not doing for yourself in the past six months because the TS management demands have taken the space where it would otherwise happen. This might be a form of physical activity, a relationship you have not invested in, a creative or professional interest that has been set aside, or simply the permission to do something unrelated to caregiving without guilt. Make one concrete plan, with a specific date and time, to do that thing in the next two weeks.

Summary

Caregiver depletion is a physiological state, not a mood, and it develops gradually through sustained high-alert caregiving that is rarely named as effort because it is simply what love requires. The specific signs, including hypervigilance, reduced enjoyment, compassion fatigue, and unexplained physical symptoms, are easy to misattribute and consistently under-attended to in TS families. Secondary stigma adds a social cost that accumulates over years and is best addressed through accurate communication and a support network that includes at least some people who understand TS. Building support before crisis makes it more available when crisis arrives. And attending to the family member's own experience is not a departure from the caregiving role; it is one of the most useful things the family member can model for the person with TS.

Conclusion Connection Is the Goal

Margot, who was eleven by the time this book was being written, went to her first overnight camp the summer after she turned ten. It was not a special needs camp. It was the ordinary kind, with cabins and a lake and competitive archery on Tuesday afternoons. She had not told anyone at camp that she had Tourette Syndrome for the first three days, partly from caution and partly from a desire to be, for a little while, just a person at camp.

On the fourth day, during a cabin activity, a cluster of tics happened during a moment of relative quiet. Another girl, not unkindly, asked what that was. Margot said: "I have Tourette Syndrome. My brain sends some extra signals sometimes. It doesn't hurt and I can't really stop it." The other girl said: "Oh, okay." And the cabin activity continued.

Margot told her mother this story on the phone that evening. Her mother, Coralie, listened to the whole thing and said: "How did that feel?" And Margot said: "Normal. It felt totally normal."

This is what the work in this book is aimed toward. Not the absence of tics. Not the resolution of the OCD or the management of the ADHD or the quiet mornings free of premonitory urge and suppression cost. Those things are worth working toward and this book has given you tools for all of them. But the goal beneath all of those tools, the one that makes the other work worth doing, is this: the person with TS in your life moving through the world with enough understanding behind them, enough preparation ahead of them, and enough warmth in the relationships that matter most, that they can say what happened in a camp cabin on an ordinary evening and call it normal.

What Changes With Knowledge

You arrived at this book in some kind of difficulty. Not necessarily crisis, but difficulty. The kind that comes from loving someone whose experience you did not yet have the information to understand. The kind that produces the car-driveway pause before going inside, the dinner table miscommunications, the misread tic attacks, the school meetings that produced goodwill and no written plan, the evenings that started wrong because nobody had designed the decompression ritual.

The information in this book does not remove the difficulty. Tourette Syndrome is a real condition with real daily implications, and no amount of reading changes the neurological reality of the premonitory urge or the suppression cost or the way the TS-Plus constellation can make a shared home genuinely complex to manage. What changes with knowledge is the quality of the difficulty. The difficulty of not understanding is different from the difficulty of understanding and still facing a challenge. The second kind is more workable. It is oriented toward action rather than confusion. It is the kind of difficulty that produces rituals and scripts and accommodation plans and treatment summaries, rather than the kind that produces silence and resentment and the slow contraction of family life around avoidances.

Knowledge changes how love is expressed. This is the most important thing this book can leave with you. The love was there before the book. The expression of it was limited by an absence of information. The book cannot provide the love. It can provide the information, and the combination produces something different from either alone.

The Relationship Is the Point

All the clinical frameworks in this book, CBIT and habit reversal training and ERP and the IEP language and the five-question media evaluation and the pre-event planning template, are instruments in service of a relationship. The relationship between the family member and the person with TS is the point of all of it. A relationship in which both people can be more fully themselves because the TS is understood rather than merely managed, and in which the TS is incorporated into a shared life rather than structured around or against.

The families who do this best are not the ones who have the least severe TS in the household. They are the ones who have invested the most consistently in the relational quality of the household, in the conversations that happen at calm moments rather than only at crisis moments, in the decompression rituals and the three-things debriefs and the timed-delay conversations and the family meetings with explicit roles and time limits. The investment is not enormous in any single instance. The cumulative effect of small, consistent investments is.

Tics are not the problem. Isolation, shame, and misunderstanding are the problem. The tics are what the family learns to live alongside. The isolation, the shame, and the misunderstanding are what the family member can genuinely, substantially, change.

What to Do This Week

Write one paragraph. It does not need to be polished or complete or entirely accurate about the future. It needs only to describe, in your own words, what kind of partner or parent or sibling you want to be for the person with TS in your life, and what one thing you will do differently this week.

Not this month. This week. Because the work of a TS family is done in weeks, and in days, and in the specific moment when the tic cluster starts in the car and the three sentences are there rather than the wrong words, and in the school meeting where the provision is named as an entitlement rather than requested as a favour, and in the decompression ritual at six o'clock that makes seven o'clock genuinely possible.

Write the paragraph. Then go do the one thing.

The relationship is worth the investment. You already knew that. You have known it since before you opened the first page.

Appendix A Glossary of Key Terms

The following terms appear throughout this book and are defined here for quick reference.

Premonitory urge. The physical sensation that builds in the body before a tic occurs, typically described as pressure, tension, or an itch that demands release. The tic resolves the urge.

Tic. A sudden, rapid, recurrent, non-rhythmic movement or sound. Tics are classified as motor (movements) or vocal (sounds), and as simple (single movement or sound) or complex (coordinated sequences of movements or sounds).

Tourette Syndrome (TS). A neurodevelopmental condition characterised by the presence of both motor and vocal tics, with onset before age 18 and duration of at least one year. Tics must not be attributable to another medical condition or substance.

Persistent tic disorder. A tic disorder involving either motor or vocal tics but not both, present for more than one year.

TS-Plus. Informal clinical term for Tourette Syndrome presenting alongside one or more co-occurring conditions, most commonly ADHD, OCD, and anxiety.

Suppression. The voluntary effort to prevent a tic from occurring. Suppression is possible for many people with TS but incurs a physiological cost and typically results in rebound when the effort is released.

Suppression rebound. The increase in tic frequency and intensity that typically follows a period of tic suppression.

ADHD (attention-deficit/hyperactivity disorder). A neurodevelopmental condition characterised by inattention, hyperactivity, and impulsivity. Present in 60 to 80 percent of people with TS.

OCD (obsessive-compulsive disorder). A condition characterised by intrusive obsessions and compulsive behaviours performed to reduce distress. In TS, OCD frequently presents with symmetry, incompleteness, and not-just-right experiences rather than the contamination and harm themes more common in OCD without TS.

Rage attacks. Episodes of explosive emotional intensity associated with TS that arise rapidly, peak briefly, and resolve, typically leaving the person with TS genuinely remorseful. Neurologically driven, not evidence of intentional aggression.

CBIT (Comprehensive Behavioral Intervention for Tics). The first-line behavioural treatment for Tourette Syndrome, consisting of habit reversal training, relaxation training, and functional intervention to identify and modify tic-maintaining environmental factors.

Habit reversal training (HRT). The core component of CBIT, in which the person with TS learns to recognise the premonitory urge and perform a competing response that is physically incompatible with the tic.

ERP (exposure and response prevention). The evidence-based treatment for OCD, in which the person is exposed to obsessional cues without performing the compulsive response, allowing habituation to occur over time.

PANS (pediatric acute-onset neuropsychiatric syndrome). A condition characterised by sudden, dramatic onset of OCD symptoms or severely restricted food intake, accompanied by acute behavioural deterioration, following an immune system activation.

PANDAS (pediatric autoimmune neuropsychiatric disorders associated with streptococcal infections). A subset of PANS in which the immune trigger is documented streptococcal infection.

Section 504 plan. A US educational accommodation plan under the Rehabilitation Act of 1973, providing equal access to education for students with documented disabilities, without requiring specially designed instruction.

IEP (Individualized Education Program). A US educational plan under the Individuals with Disabilities Education Act, providing specially designed instruction for students whose disability adversely affects educational performance.

EHC plan (Education, Health and Care plan). The UK equivalent of the IEP, available in England under the Children and Families Act 2014 for students whose needs cannot be met through standard school-based support.

Coprolalia. The involuntary vocalisation of obscene or taboo words. A tic affecting approximately 10 to 20 percent of people with TS.

Copropraxia. The involuntary performance of obscene gestures. A tic that is less common than coprolalia.

Family accommodation. The term used in OCD research for the ways family members adjust their behaviour to manage OCD symptoms. Higher accommodation is associated with greater OCD severity.

Appendix B Recommended Resources

The following organisations provide reliable, research-grounded information about Tourette Syndrome, tic disorders, and the related conditions described in this book. All resources listed have been selected for accuracy and currency.

Tourette Association of America (tourette.org). The primary advocacy and information organisation for TS in the United States. Provides family guides, school accommodation resources, a CBIT provider directory, research summaries, and support group information. The family resources section is specifically designed for parents and partners.

New Jersey Center for Tourette Syndrome and Associated Disorders (njcts.org). Provides educator and parent resources with particular strength in school advocacy and the TS-Plus clinical profile. The TS Parents Online section includes practical guidance for school navigation.

Tourettes Action UK (tourettes.org.uk). The primary UK advocacy organisation. Provides resources calibrated to the UK educational and healthcare system, including EHCP guidance and UK-specific practitioner referrals.

CDC Tourette Syndrome pages (cdc.gov/tourette). Provides epidemiological data, evidence summaries, and public information that is free from commercial interest. Useful for providing to healthcare providers unfamiliar with TS who prefer government sources.

PANDAS Network (pandasnetwork.org). Provides the most accessible family-oriented information on PANS and PANDAS, including a diagnostic overview, provider directory, and support group listings.

TicHelper (tichelper.com). An online platform offering computerised CBIT content for families in areas without access to

CBIT-trained practitioners. The underlying approach is evidence-based and the platform has been studied in clinical trials.

Tourette Association of America CBIT provider directory. Available through tourette.org, this directory lists practitioners who have received CBIT training. Telehealth entries are available for families without local access.

Appendix C Communication Scripts Reference Card

The following scripts are condensed from Chapter 5 for quick reference. They are designed to be read aloud, memorised, and available before they are needed.

During a tic attack or tic cluster at home or in public. Say: "I see you. Take what space you need. I am right here." Do not pull over, do not ask questions, do not provide additional commentary. Return to ordinary activity after delivering the three sentences.

After an acute episode, before processing. Say: "That looked hard. I am here whenever you want to talk about it. No rush." Then wait until the person with TS initiates. Do not follow up within the first hour.

When OCD reassurance is requested. Say: "I can hear this feels hard right now. That sounds like OCD looking for certainty it will not get from me. You have handled this before." Do not provide the reassurance. Do not refuse angrily. Acknowledge and redirect.

Opening a treatment conversation. Say: "I have been reading about [specific treatment]. I want to understand it better. Would you be willing to read about it with me?" Frame as shared inquiry rather than proposal.

Explaining TS to someone who does not understand it. Say: "They have a condition called Tourette Syndrome. Imagine having an itch you physically could not stop scratching, even if you wanted to, even if scratching made people stare. That is what it feels like before a tic. The tic is the scratch." Use the itch-and-scratch metaphor as the primary explanatory tool.

Responding to a stranger after a tic in public. Say: "He has Tourette Syndrome. It is a tic. He cannot control it." Then resume ordinary activity. For persistent strangers: "I understand you are surprised. He has a neurological condition. We are fine, thank you."

When a family member provides OCD-related misinformation. Correct the specific statement, not the general framework. Say: "Actually, the research shows that the tics are involuntary. The part that helps is understanding the premonitory urge, which is the physical sensation that comes before. It is something like an itch." Then use the itch-and-scratch explanation.

Appendix D School Accommodation Request Template

The following template is designed to be personalised and submitted to a school or educational authority. Replace bracketed text with the relevant details. Review with a treating clinician before submission where possible.

[Parent/Guardian name]

[Date]

[School name, administrator name, and role]

Subject: Accommodation Request for [Student name], [Grade/Year], [Diagnosis]

I am writing to request formal educational accommodations for my child, [student name], who has been diagnosed with Tourette Syndrome and [list TS-Plus diagnoses if applicable] by [clinician name and credential] on [date]. A copy of the clinical documentation is attached.

[Student name]'s condition substantially limits their ability to [specify: concentrate, communicate, participate in standardised assessment, or other relevant activity]. Under [Section 504 of the Rehabilitation Act of 1973, the Americans with Disabilities Act, the Children and Families Act 2014, or the Disability Standards for Education 2005, as applicable], the school is required to provide reasonable accommodations to ensure equal access to education.

I am requesting the following specific accommodations.

First: [Accommodation 1, e.g., preferential seating at the end of a row or near an exit, to allow for quiet tic release without distracting classmates.]

Second: [Accommodation 2, e.g., permission to take brief movement breaks of two to five minutes when tic pressure becomes unmanageable, without penalty.]

Third: [Accommodation 3, e.g., extended time of 50 percent on all timed assessments, to account for the cognitive load of tic management during high-pressure tasks.]

Fourth: [Accommodation 4 if applicable, e.g., access to a quiet room for standardised testing.]

Fifth: [Accommodation 5 if applicable, e.g., modified homework load on days of elevated tic severity, as documented by parent communication.]

I request that these accommodations be documented in a written plan, reviewed by all teaching staff who work with [student name], and reviewed at minimum annually. I am available to meet to discuss these accommodations at your earliest convenience.

Please respond in writing within [ten working days, or the statutory period applicable in your jurisdiction].

[Parent/Guardian signature and contact information]

Note for UK families. If requesting an EHC plan assessment, the opening of this letter should state: "I am writing to formally request that the local authority conduct an Education, Health and Care needs assessment for my child [name], under Section 36 of the Children and Families Act 2014." The local authority is legally required to respond within six weeks.

Note for Australian families. Reference the Disability Standards for Education 2005 and the school's obligations under the Disability Discrimination Act 1992. Request that the reasonable adjustment be documented in writing.

Appendix E CBIT and Treatment Provider Questions

The following questions are designed to be brought to clinical appointments. They are grouped by provider type.

For a neurologist or movement disorder specialist.

What is the current recommended first-line treatment for Tourette Syndrome, and has it been offered to us? What is the expected trajectory for tic severity in this patient over the next five years? What TS-Plus conditions have been formally assessed, and which require additional evaluation? What medication, if any, would you recommend at this stage, and what would you expect it to achieve? If medication is recommended, what are the most likely side effects and how will they be monitored? At what point would you consider a referral to a CBIT-trained practitioner? Is deep brain stimulation evaluation relevant for this patient, and if so, where would that evaluation happen?

For a CBIT therapist at an initial consultation.

What specific competing responses do you expect to develop for this patient's primary tics? What is the family member's role in the treatment, and what specific changes should we make at home? How will the functional assessment be used to modify our daily routine? What does the evidence suggest about outcomes for someone with this patient's tic profile? How many sessions do you typically recommend, and what does maintenance look like after the intensive phase? Is there anything about this patient's TS-Plus profile that would modify the standard CBIT approach?

For a psychiatrist managing TS-Plus conditions.

Which of this patient's conditions is currently most impairing and should be the primary treatment target? If OCD is present, has exposure and response prevention been considered or implemented? What is the evidence base for the medication you are recommending, specifically for TS-related OCD or ADHD rather than the general population? What is the expected timeline for seeing a meaningful response to the current treatment? How are the tics and the TS-Plus conditions interacting, and does treating one tend to affect the other? Is there a family accommodation pattern that is maintaining the OCD, and if so, how should we begin addressing it?

For a school meeting (IEP, 504, or EHC plan review).

Which of the requested accommodations will be included in the written plan, and which will not, and what is the reason for any exclusion? Who is responsible for ensuring each accommodation is implemented, and what is the process if it is not? How will the plan be communicated to all teaching staff who work with this student? What is the review timeline, and who initiates the review? If the student's needs change between reviews, what is the process for requesting an amendment? What is the escalation pathway if we believe the plan is not being followed?

References

Baldermann, J. C., Schuller, T., Huys, D., Timmermann, L., Jessen, F., Visser-Vandewalle, V., & Kuhn, J. (2016). Deep brain stimulation for Tourette-syndrome: A systematic review and meta-analysis. Brain Stimulation, 9(2), 296-304. https://doi.org/10.1016/j.brs.2015.11.005

Barkley, R. A. (2006). Attention-deficit hyperactivity disorder: A handbook for diagnosis and treatment (3rd ed.). Guilford Press.

Bloch, M. H., & Leckman, J. F. (2009). Clinical course of Tourette syndrome. Journal of Psychosomatic Research, 67(6), 497-501. https://doi.org/10.1016/j.jpsychores.2009.09.002

Budman, C. L., Bruun, R. D., Park, K. S., & Olson, M. E. (2000). Explosive outbursts in children with Tourette's disorder. Journal of the American Academy of Child and Adolescent Psychiatry, 39(10), 1270-1276. https://doi.org/10.1097/00004583-200010000-00013

Chang, K., Frankovich, J., Cooperstock, M., Cunningham, M. W., Latimer, M. E., Murphy, T. K., Pasternack, M., Thienemann, M., Williams, K., Walter, J., & Swedo, S. E. (2015). Clinical evaluation of youth with pediatric acute-onset neuropsychiatric syndrome (PANS): Recommendations from the 2013 PANS Consensus Conference. Journal of Child and Adolescent Psychopharmacology, 25(1), 3-13. https://doi.org/10.1089/cap.2014.0084

Conelea, C. A., & Woods, D. W. (2008). The influence of contextual factors on tic expression in Tourette's syndrome: A review. Journal of Psychosomatic Research, 65(5), 487-496. https://doi.org/10.1016/j.jpsychores.2008.04.010

Conelea, C. A., Carter, A. C., & Freeman, J. B. (2013). Sensory over-responsivity in a sample of children seeking treatment for anxiety. Journal of Developmental and Behavioral Pediatrics, 35(7), 484-492. https://doi.org/10.1097/DBP.0b013e3182a39a9a

Cooperstock, M. S., Swedo, S. E., Pasternack, M. S., Murphy, T. K., & PANS/PANDAS Consortium. (2017). Clinical management of pediatric acute-onset neuropsychiatric syndrome: Part III, treatment and prevention of infections. Journal of Child and Adolescent Psychopharmacology, 27(7), 594-606. https://doi.org/10.1089/cap.2016.0151

Corrigan, P. W., Druss, B. G., & Perlick, D. A. (2016). The impact of mental illness stigma on seeking and participating in mental health care. Psychological Science in the Public Interest, 15(2), 37-70. https://doi.org/10.1177/1529100615583500

Eddy, C. M., Rizzo, R., Gulisano, M., Agodi, A., Barchitta, M., Calì, P., Robertson, M. M., & Cavanna, A. E. (2011). Quality of life in young people with Tourette syndrome: A controlled study. Journal of Neurology, 258(2), 291-301. https://doi.org/10.1007/s00415-010-5754-6

U.S. Department of Education, Office for Civil Rights. (2023). Protecting students with disabilities. https://www2.ed.gov/about/offices/list/ocr/504faq.html

Findley, D. B. (2001). Characteristics of tic disorders. In D. W. Woods & R. G. Miltenberger (Eds.), Tic disorders, trichotillomania, and other repetitive behavior disorders (pp. 53-100). Kluwer Academic.

Tourette Syndrome Association International Consortium for Genetics. (2007). Genome scan for Tourette disorder in affected-sibling-pair and multigenerational families.

American Journal of Human Genetics, 80(2), 265-272. https://doi.org/10.1086/511052

Ghosh, D., Rajan, P. V., Das, D., Datta, P., Rothner, A. D., & Erenberg, G. (2014). Sleep disorders in children with Tourette syndrome. Pediatric Neurology, 51(1), 31-35. https://doi.org/10.1016/j.pediatrneurol.2014.03.017

Harvey, A. G. (2002). A cognitive model of insomnia. Behaviour Research and Therapy, 40(8), 869-893. https://doi.org/10.1016/S0005-7967(01)00061-4

Himle, M. B., Woods, D. W., Conelea, C. A., Bauer, C. C., & Rice, K. A. (2007). Investigating the effects of tic suppression on premonitory urge ratings in children and adolescents with Tourette's syndrome. Behaviour Research and Therapy, 45(12), 2964-2976. https://doi.org/10.1016/j.brat.2006.12.007

Himle, M. B., & Woods, D. W. (2005). An experimental evaluation of tic suppression and the tic rebound effect. Behaviour Research and Therapy, 43(11), 1443-1451. https://doi.org/10.1016/j.brat.2004.11.002

Tourette Association of America. (2023). School accommodations for students with Tourette syndrome. https://tourette.org

Tourette Association of America. (2023). Parent and family resources: Living with Tourette syndrome. https://tourette.org/about-tourette/overview/living-tourette-syndrome/parent-family-resources/

Jankovic, J., Jimenez-Shahed, J., & Brown, L. W. (2010). A randomised, double-blind, placebo-controlled study of topiramate in the treatment of Tourette syndrome. Journal of Neurology, Neurosurgery and Psychiatry, 81(1), 70-73. https://doi.org/10.1136/jnnp.2009.185348

Khalifa, N., & von Knorring, A. L. (2005). Tourette syndrome and other tic disorders in a total population of children: Clinical assessment and background. Acta Paediatrica, 94(11), 1608-1614. https://doi.org/10.1111/j.1651-2227.2005.tb01837.x

Leckman, J. F., Walker, D. E., & Cohen, D. J. (1993). Premonitory urges in Tourette's syndrome. American Journal of Psychiatry, 150(1), 98-102. https://doi.org/10.1176/ajp.150.1.98

Leckman, J. F., Zhang, H., Vitale, A., Lahnin, F., Lynch, K., Bondi, C., Kim, Y. S., & Peterson, B. S. (1998). Course of tic severity in Tourette syndrome: The first two decades. Pediatrics, 102(1), 14-19. https://doi.org/10.1542/peds.102.1.14

Majeske, M., Brar, H., Wexler, L., & Hall, C. (2018). Psychological distress in parents of children with Tourette syndrome. Journal of Child Neurology, 33(7), 461-467. https://doi.org/10.1177/0883073818758692

March, J. S., Frances, A., Carpenter, D., & Kahn, D. A. (1997). The expert consensus guideline series: Treatment of obsessive-compulsive disorder. Journal of Clinical Psychiatry, 58(Suppl 4), 1-72.

McCabe, M. P., McDonald, E., Deeks, A. A., Vowels, L. M., & Cobain, M. J. (2003). The impact of multiple sclerosis on sexuality and relationships. Journal of Sex Research, 40(2), 154-162. https://doi.org/10.1080/00224490309552178

Miguel, E. C., do Rosario-Campos, M. C., Prado, H. S., do Valle, R., Rauch, S. L., Coffey, B. J., Baer, L., Savage, C. R., O'Sullivan, R. L., Jenike, M. A., & Leckman, J. F. (2000). Sensory phenomena in obsessive-compulsive disorder and Tourette's disorder. Journal of Clinical Psychiatry, 61(2), 150-156. https://doi.org/10.4088/jcp.v61n0213

Murphy, T. K., Lewin, A. B., Storch, E. A., Stock, S., & American Academy of Child and Adolescent Psychiatry Committee on Quality Issues. (2013). Practice parameter for the assessment and treatment of children and adolescents with tic disorders. Journal of the American Academy of Child and Adolescent Psychiatry, 52(12), 1341-1359. https://doi.org/10.1016/j.jaac.2013.09.015

Tourette Syndrome Study Group. (2002). Treatment of ADHD in children with tics: A randomized controlled trial. Neurology, 58(4), 527-536. https://doi.org/10.1212/WNL.58.4.527

Van Noppen, B., & Steketee, G. (2009). Testing a conceptual model of patient and family predictors of obsessive compulsive disorder (OCD) symptoms. Behaviour Research and Therapy, 47(1), 18-25. https://doi.org/10.1016/j.brat.2008.10.005

Piacentini, J., Woods, D. W., Scahill, L., Wilhelm, S., Peterson, A. L., Chang, S., Ginsburg, G. S., Deckersbach, T., Dziura, J., Levi-Pearl, S., & Walkup, J. T. (2010). Behavior therapy for children with Tourette disorder: A randomized controlled trial. JAMA, 303(19), 1929-1937. https://doi.org/10.1001/jama.2010.607

Pringsheim, T., Okun, M. S., Muller-Vahl, K., Martino, D., Jankovic, J., Cavanna, A. E., Woods, D. W., Robinson, M., Jarvie, E., Roessner, V., Oskoui, M., Holler-Managan, Y., & Piacentini, J. (2019). Practice guideline recommendations summary: Treatment of tics in people with Tourette syndrome and chronic tic disorders. Neurology, 92(19), 896-906. https://doi.org/10.1212/WNL.0000000000007466

Pringsheim, T., Ganos, C., McGuire, J. F., Hedderly, T., Woods, D., Gilbert, D. L., Piacentini, J., & Cavanna, A. E. (2021). Rapid onset functional tic-like behaviors in young females during the COVID-19 pandemic. Movement Disorders, 36(12), 2707-2713. https://doi.org/10.1002/mds.28778

Ricketts, E. J., Goetz, A. R., Capriotti, M. R., Bauer, C. C., Brei, N. G., Himle, M. B., Espil, F. M., Snorrason, I., Aldridge, J. W., Woods, D. W., & Zinner, S. H. (2016). A randomized waitlist-controlled pilot trial of voice over Internet protocol-delivered behavior therapy for youth with chronic tic disorders. Journal of Telemedicine and Telecare, 22(3), 153-162. https://doi.org/10.1177/1357633X15593192

Robertson, M. M., Eapen, V., Singer, H. S., Martino, D., Scharf, J. M., Paschou, P., Roessner, V., Woods, D. W., Hariz, M., Cath, D. C., Ludolph, A., Stern, J. S., & Leckman, J. F. (2017). Gilles de la Tourette syndrome. Nature Reviews Disease Primers, 3, 16097. https://doi.org/10.1038/nrdp.2016.97

Sharpe, D., & Rossiter, L. (2002). Siblings of children with a chronic illness: A meta-analysis. Journal of Pediatric Psychology, 27(8), 699-710. https://doi.org/10.1093/jpepsy/27.8.699

Snider, L. A., & Swedo, S. E. (2004). PANDAS: Current status and directions for research. Molecular Psychiatry, 9(10), 900-907. https://doi.org/10.1038/sj.mp.4001542

Storch, E. A., Murphy, T. K., Chase, R. M., Keeley, M., Goodman, W. K., Murray, M., & Geffken, G. R. (2007). Peer victimization in youth with Tourette's syndrome and chronic tic disorder: Relations with tic severity and internalizing symptoms. Journal of Psychopathology and Behavioral Assessment, 29(4), 211-219. https://doi.org/10.1007/s10862-006-9050-0

Storch, E. A., Geffken, G. R., Merlo, L. J., Jacob, M. L., Murphy, T. K., Goodman, W. K., Larson, M. J., Fernandez, M., & Grabill, K. (2007). Family accommodation in pediatric obsessive-compulsive disorder. Journal of Clinical Child and Adolescent Psychology, 36(2), 207-216. https://doi.org/10.1080/15374410701277929

Storch, E. A., Lewin, A. B., Geffken, G. R., Morgan, J. R., & Murphy, T. K. (2010). The role of comorbid disruptive behavior in the clinical expression of pediatric obsessive-compulsive disorder. Behaviour Research and Therapy, 48(12), 1173-1179. https://doi.org/10.1016/j.brat.2010.08.007

Sukhodolsky, D. G., Scahill, L., Zhang, H., Peterson, B. S., King, R. A., Lombroso, P. J., Katsovich, L., Findley, D., & Leckman, J. F. (2003). Disruptive behavior in children with Tourette's syndrome: Association with ADHD comorbidity, tic severity, and functional impairment. Journal of the American Academy of Child and Adolescent Psychiatry, 42(1), 98-105. https://doi.org/10.1097/00004583-200301000-00016

Whittingham, K., Wee, D., & Boyd, R. (2011). Systematic review of the efficacy of parenting interventions for children with cerebral palsy. Child: Care, Health and Development, 37(4), 475-483. https://doi.org/10.1111/j.1365-2214.2011.01212.x

Wilhelm, S., Peterson, A. L., Piacentini, J., Woods, D. W., Deckersbach, T., Sukhodolsky, D. G., Chang, S., Liu, H., Dziura, J., Walkup, J. T., & Scahill, L. (2012). Randomized trial of behavior therapy for adults with Tourette syndrome. Archives of General Psychiatry, 69(8), 795-803. https://doi.org/10.1001/archgenpsychiatry.2011.1528

Woods, D. W., Piacentini, J., Himle, M. B., & Chang, S. (2005). Premonitory urge for tics scale (PUTS): Initial psychometric results and examination of the premonitory urge phenomenon in youths with tic disorders. Journal of

Developmental and Behavioral Pediatrics, 26(6), 397-403. https://doi.org/10.1097/00004703-200512000-00001

Woods, D. W., Piacentini, J. C., & Walkup, J. T. (Eds.). (2007). Treating Tourette syndrome and tic disorders: A guide for practitioners. Guilford Press.

Zito, R. (2025). When you're (not) the stereotype: Coprolalia stigma in the lives of adults with Tourette syndrome. Deviant Behavior. https://doi.org/10.1080/01639625.2025.2531145

Made in the USA
Monee, IL
04 November 2026

67387164R00085